Prais

"Debby Herbenick says it herself... ...lled with prompts, real world examp... ...ions about sexuality between adults and the kids in their care. No topic is taboo. No question is unaskable. This phenomenal resource offers guidance for talking with kids of any age about how to value themselves, how to value others, and how to create a world that uplifts rather than tears down. It's a must-have for every adult who's ever asked, 'How do I talk with my kid about that?'"

—Al Vernacchio, author of *For Goodness Sex*

"This is the book parents and caregivers need to feel more confident raising kids in today's tech-, sex-, and social media–saturated world. Loaded with practical tips and helpful scripts, backed by research, this is a must-read for becoming an askable, informed adult to young people."

—Melissa Pintor Carnagey, LBSW, founder and lead educator at Sex Positive Families and author of *Sex Positive Talks to Have with Kids*

"As a college health and STD expert, I regularly see the challenging consequences of hormone-, alcohol-, and/or drug-fueled impulsive choices. These topics are frankly awkward or uncomfortable for most, but parents need to know what *Yes, Your Kid* reveals. This book takes parent sex ed to a whole new level with practical dialog, frank discussions, and especially the extra layer of unexpected potential legal ramifications."

—Jill Grimes, MD, FAAFP, author of *Seductive Delusions* and *The Ultimate College Student Health Handbook*

"Parents need not dread 'the talk' about sex any longer. In *Yes, Your Kid*, Debby Herbenick provides us with the skills we need to become the ultimate 'askable parent' when it comes to sexuality. Full of wisdom, cutting-edge research, and practical advice, *Yes, Your Kid* is an essential read for parents, educators, and anyone else trying to support our teens' sexual health in a complex and increasingly digital world."

—Ina Park, MD, author of *Strange Bedfellows*

"There is a lot of new, sometimes scary, ground to cover as we do our best to prepare young people to have healthy and fulfilling relationships, explore their sexuality in safe and enjoyable ways, and avoid causing or experiencing sexual trauma. In *Yes, Your Kid*, Herbenick, a nationally respected sexuality researcher, college professor, and mom presents facts, real-world insights, and advice that is practical, judgment-free, and wrapped in compassion. Her coauthors share legal insights that every teen and young adult should understand. *Yes, Your Kid* should be the trusted resource for all parents who care about guiding their tweens and teens toward healthy exploration of relationships and sexuality. Some of it may seem shocking, but so is the sexual content our kids are growing up with. Every page is deeply rooted in facts, research, and the unique insights of the authors who work with college students every day. Read it cover to cover, then come back to it as a reference book to address each of the issues at the right time for your child and your family. Parenting teens and young adults involves a lot of tough talks, and *Yes, Your Kid* is a perfect guidebook for talking about relationships and sexual health."

—Melisa Holmes, MD, FACOG, pediatric and adolescent gynecologist, mother of three, cofounder of Girlology, and author of *You-ology*

"*Yes, Your Kid* is an exceptionally well-researched and well-written text addressing the challenging issues facing our young people. Using a conversational approach, Debby Herbenick and her coauthors do not shy away from unpacking difficult and yet crucial topics such as consent, puberty, sexual and reproductive health, sex and technology, pornography, and many more. *Yes, Your Kid* is the book I wish I had had when my three daughters were growing up as it provides parents with the language and the tools to broach these topics with confidence and knowledge. A must-have book for all parents and carers."

—Jayneen Sanders, author of *My Body! What I Say Goes!* and *Let's Talk About Body Boundaries, Consent, and Respect*

"*Yes, Your Kid* is a must-read for every parent that wants to protect and empower their child. Media and the internet are having a profound impact on situations teens are facing with peers and those wishing to exploit. To protect their kids, parents must inform themselves and educate their children. Dr. Herbenick clearly explains the changing sexual landscape in our country, and gives practical advice on how to talk with youth at each stage to equip them in protecting themselves while simultaneously building strong, caring, and mutually protective relationships. Special attention is given to neurodiversity, pornography, the increase in nonconsensual rough sex, and resources. Parents, teachers, caregivers, and coaches: Do yourself a favor and read this book! Equip yourselves to equip your teens."

—Dr. Tina Schermer Sellers, PhD, LMFT, CST-S, author of *Shameless Parenting*

"Parenting today is not for the faint of heart—and that's where *Yes, Your Kid* comes in to save the day. With common-sense and research-based advice about how to talk to kids and teens about sexuality, it's the resource parents need right now. With discussions around sexuality so different from when today's parents were kids, and so many changes in technology, we all need more information than what we learned in sex ed class so long ago. Sometimes our Gen Z kids use terms around sexual identity many Gen X and even Millennial parents have never heard of! Our kids need better information about sex, but many parents just don't know what to say—that's where *Yes, Your Kid* can help. An engaging and very helpful read."

—Jean M. Twenge, PhD, author of *Generations*

YES,
YOUR
KID

Also by Debby Herbenick, PhD

Because It Feels Good: A Woman's Guide to Sexual Pleasure and Satisfaction

Sex Made Easy: Your Awkward Questions Answered—
for Better, Smarter, Amazing Sex

Read My Lips: A Complete Guide to the Vagina and Vulva
(with Vanessa Schick)

The Coregasm Workout: The Revolutionary Method
for Better Sex Through Exercise

Great in Bed (with Grant Stoddard)

YES, YOUR KID

What Parents Need to Know About Today's Teens and Sex

DEBBY HERBENICK, PhD

with Kristina W. Supler, Esq., and Susan C. Stone, Esq.

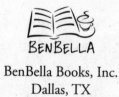

BENBELLA

BenBella Books, Inc.
Dallas, TX

BenBella Books, Inc.
10440 N. Central Expressway
Suite 800
Dallas, TX 75231
benbellabooks.com
Send feedback to feedback@benbellabooks.com

BenBella is a federally registered trademark.

Printed in the United States of America
10 9 8 7 6 5 4 3 2 1

Library of Congress Control Number: 2023016163
ISBN 9781637743805 (trade paperback)
ISBN 9781637743812 (electronic)

Editing by Leah Wilson
Copyediting by Scott Calamar
Proofreading by Jennifer Canzoneri and Karen Wise
Indexing by Amy Murphy
Text design and composition by PerfecType, Nashville, TN
Cover design by Brigid Pearson
Printed by Lake Book Manufacturing

To every parent who has pulled me aside at a birthday party or soccer game or messaged me with questions about sexuality.

To my students, who have trusted me with their ups and downs.

And to Cindy and John, for modeling what it means to be askable parents.
—D.H.

We dedicate this book to our clients. We are honored to serve you.
—K.S. & S.S.

CONTENTS

INTRODUCTION

One morning last spring, I woke to the sound of raindrops lightly pitter-pattering against our windows. I stayed in bed for several minutes, relishing the quiet and anticipating the sounds of our children who would soon be up and about, getting ready for school. Then I reached over to the nightstand to find my phone and check the time. Overnight, my screen had filled with messages from a childhood friend.* "I'm sorry to bother you but I need your help!" read the first message, sent after midnight. The messages that followed described how my friend and her teenage daughter have an understanding that allows my friend to check her teen's phone on occasion, which she said she had done only rarely because previous checks had turned up nothing of concern. This time, however, she came across a detailed text exchange between her daughter and her daughter's boyfriend in which they'd discussed how much they both like when he slaps her during sex. "I didn't even know they were having sex," my friend wrote. "I wish she would have come to me first. But mostly I'm freaking out about him slapping my daughter, which scares me. She's doing great in school, she has friends. Between *Fifty Shades of Grey* and internet porn, have times just changed? Am I overreacting? What should I say to her?"

---

* Names and identifying details of friends, students, and clients have been changed throughout the book. In some instances, composite examples have been created for anonymity.

1

My friend reached out not because we are especially close—in fact, it had been several years since we'd seen one another in person—but because she was surprised by what she learned about her daughter's sexual experiences and not sure where else to turn for well-informed, nonjudgmental help. Perhaps you've found yourself in similar shoes, trying to figure out how to address a challenging parenting conundrum while staying close and connected with your child (and not wanting to risk seeming out of touch or overly panicked).

As a sexuality researcher and educator, it is literally my job to understand human sexual behavior, including the sexual lives of teenagers and young adults. I'm a professor at the Indiana University School of Public Health, where I lead the National Survey of Sexual Health and Behavior—a large US nationally representative survey that tracks Americans' sex lives from adolescence through advanced age. I also teach college courses in sexual and reproductive health, which means I'm surrounded by students who keep me current on new sexual trends and terms. And, as a mom, I love hearing my own children's questions and curiosities about the world, including about puberty, pregnancy, dating, sexual behavior, and love. Even at young ages, they've asked both difficult questions ("What if someone becomes pregnant but they don't want to be pregnant?") and funny questions ("When you and dad put your vagina and penis together to make us, did you have to be naked? What day was it on?").

But it's not only children who are full of questions. People of all ages have questions and concerns about sexual feelings, attractions, and their health, regardless of age. Because of my work, I often hear what's on the minds of friends, family, colleagues, students, and readers—many of whom are parents. I'm asked questions like:

- "Our daughter is in kindergarten, and we haven't yet talked about vaginas or penises or how babies are made. Where should we start and what should we say?"

- "When should we talk with our son about pornography? We don't want to introduce the idea if he hasn't yet seen pornography, but we also don't want to wait until it's too late to talk about it."
- "My sixth grader asked me to buy her a vibrator. I want to normalize masturbation, but this also seems far too young for a sex toy. Is it?"
- "How do I prepare my transgender son for getting their period, when they don't want to even think about having a uterus or vagina?"
- "Why are so many kids coming out as LGBTQ+ these days? What's changed?"
- "I overheard my sixteen-year-old talking with a friend, and it sounded like one of them may have nude pictures of a classmate on their phone. I'm worried that he could get expelled from school or in trouble with the law. What should I do?"
- "My teenager was messaged by a stranger on Instagram who offered to pay her $200 for nude pictures of herself. I'm glad she felt she could tell me, and she's already blocked him, but I'm still in shock. Help!"

Fielding questions from parents trying to navigate conversations with their child around bodies or sexuality is typical in my world, and it has been since I began working in this subject area more than twenty years ago. Yet, so much about sex has changed in the past decade that the questions themselves are now considerably different. Technology has shifted in ways that were unimaginable back when many of us were watching *The Jetsons* and other cartoonish visions of the future. With changes in technology came changes in sex, including how people meet, date, flirt, and explore their sexuality. These days, teens and young adults aren't just grappling with decisions about if or when to become sexually active, but also whether they should send nude images to a classmate, fully aware that digital footprints can last forever. Alarmingly, the decision of whether to send a sexy image often comes as early as age nine or ten. Some changes have been positive (more effective forms of birth control, greater social acceptance of LGBTQ+ people) and others frightening (adults approaching teens online, cyberbullying, political backlash around LGBTQ+ rights).

Having been raised with very little information about sex, it feels meaningful for me to support families on their parenting journey. Indeed, while writing this book, it dawned on me that I was writing the book that I wish my parents had had at home when I was growing up—a book that would have offered my parents the skills, information, and confidence to talk with me about puberty, relationships, and sexuality. Like many of us, my childhood home was marked by silence when it came to these topics. I had to figure out most things on my own, including what a menstrual period was and what the kids at school meant by "first base" and "second base" (it turned out not to be kickball). And when I wanted to switch from pads to tampons to make swim practice more feasible, I secretly rode my bike far beyond my quiet suburban neighborhood in Miami, Florida— against my family's explicitly stated rules—so that I could buy tampons at a convenience store. Although I was a kid who generally followed the rules, in this case breaking the rules seemed easier than breaking my family's culture of silence.

Having parents who felt comfortable and equipped to talk with me about bodies and sexuality would have made my adolescence a lot less confusing. However, their silence shaped me into the sexuality researcher and educator I am today: a person who believes in offering people fact-based information to support them in understanding their bodies and sexual feelings and in navigating their choices. I think it would have meant a great deal to my parents if someone had said, "Talking about puberty and sexuality may feel awkward at first, but you can do this. Here's how." And this book aims to do exactly that, by providing up-to-date information about some of the most pressing sexuality issues facing young people today, as well as easy-to-follow tips for having even the most difficult conversations with your child.

PARENTS' ROLE IN SEX EDUCATION

Parents and caregivers are always teaching their children about sex, even when they don't realize it. Young people learn from observing how those around them talk about their own and others' bodies and show affection, as well as when they laugh or cringe while watching certain kinds of movie and television scenes. They notice when adults directly answer (or nervously sidestep) questions about pregnancy, marriage, divorce, sexy song lyrics, or unfamiliar terms that seem to have something to do with sex. Gender roles are understood from the media they are exposed to as well as by observing who in their family cooks meals, clears the table, takes out the trash, works at a paid job, or helps with homework.

The question, then, is not whether you should teach your child about sex, bodies, and gender; you're already doing that. Instead, it's about what you may be conveying to your child, whether through words or silence. Ask yourself:

- To what extent does your child think of you as approachable or easy to talk to when it comes to questions about sex? Are you someone your child can ask questions of without feeling shamed or blamed?
- In what ways do your family's comments and conversations about sex, gender, and relationships reflect your family's values, such as respect, acceptance, care, compassion, gender equity, responsibility, or doing the right thing?
- How do your conversations with your child reflect the realities of what sex is like today and what they need to know to feel supported and thrive in today's world?
- Does your family communicate about sex, gender, and relationships in ways that are likely to help your child create consensual, caring, and pleasurable experiences if or when they decide to have sex?

If your answers to some of these questions are marked by doubt or uncertainty, you're not alone. Many parents of teens and young adults didn't grow up with smartphones, social media, or widely accessible pornography. This is new territory! And it is shifting all the time. Yet, in a recent US nationally representative survey, 60 percent of eighteen- to twenty-four-year-olds said they'd never had a conversation with their parents about their family's values around sex.[1] And when it comes to talking about sex, studies find that teenagers want their parents to say something rather than nothing (though they could do with fewer fear tactics).

That so few parents talk with their children about sex is unfortunate. After all, parents are the single biggest influence on their teens' choices about sex—decisions such as when and with whom to become sexually active, the kind(s) of partners they date or hook up with, and even whether they use condoms or other forms of birth control. Teens whose parents have talked with them about safer sex tend to make safer choices, including postponing becoming sexually active with a partner and being more likely to use condoms or other forms of birth control when they eventually have intercourse.[2] Yet, it can be difficult for parents to figure out how much to say and when—especially when efforts to start a conversation are met with awkward silence, eye rolls, or a dismissive "I already know that." Teenagers are experts at appearing bored on the outside, but that doesn't mean they aren't interested in what their parents have to say. They may just feel uncomfortable talking about sex. It's important to talk with them anyway.

THIS BOOK IS FOR YOU

Yes, Your Kid is meant to support you in talking with your child about a broad range of sexuality topics—especially those topics that, at first glance, might seem relevant to some *other* child, but not your own. Even if you suspect your child is too young, not yet interested in sex, or more focused on school or sports than dating, this book is still for you. All children benefit from learning age- and developmentally appropriate sexuality information. Although the focus of this book is on tweens through the college years, even parents of young children will find relevant tips throughout. If you'd like to grow more comfortable and confident talking within your family about sexuality topics, you'll find concrete advice for becoming a more askable, approachable parent. Take what works, shape it to align with your family's values, and leave what doesn't fit. *Yes, Your Kid* is full of fact-based information on varied topics to support conversations at different stages of development.

Even if you already feel comfortable talking about sexuality basics with your child, you have likely realized that sex has changed dramatically since you were growing up, making updated information vital for family conversations. Consider *Yes, Your Kid* your sex education catch-up. Most parents have no idea what sex is like for young people today. You can't know what you don't know, so this book is here to fill in those gaps. What you do with that information is up to you. Between sexting, easily accessible pornography, social media, and a rapid increase in rough sex practices among teens and young adults, the evidence is clear: young people need sexuality education that reflects the kinds of sex they are seeing on screens and contemplating (or already having) in real life. And, as many schools aren't allowed to teach about some of the most basic sexual health topics (STIs, birth control, sexual orientation), parents are left with a lot of ground to cover. To help with that, I've included sample conversations and up-to-date information, and I've suggested ways that parents can band together to create community-based sexuality education rather than always going it alone.

As middle schools, high schools, and colleges create more policies that address sexting, image-based sexual abuse (sometimes referred to as "revenge porn"), sexual harassment, and sexual assault, it's also important for families to talk with their children about these school rules (as well as other state/province and federal laws). To support parents with these conversations, *Yes, Your Kid* also highlights real-life case examples from Kristina Supler and Susan Stone, attorneys who have worked nationwide on hundreds of sexual misconduct and sexual assault cases. Some have been criminal cases and others have been campus misconduct cases involving students in elementary school (yes, believe it or not), middle school, high school, college, and graduate school. A subset of these have been tried simultaneously in both criminal courts and campus proceedings.

Kristina, Susan, and I first connected because some of the cases they had worked on brought them to find my research on changing sexual norms—specifically the rapid rise in both consensual and nonconsensual rough sex practices. We shared what we were each seeing in our respective professional spheres and discussed the stark realities of the sexual choices young people now have to navigate *(Do I send them nudes? Will they lose interest in me if I'm not more sexually adventurous?)*, as well as how different these realities are from the way sex is presented in young people's very limited school-based sex education. It became apparent to us that young people aren't being adequately prepared for the world they're growing up in.

After these initial conversations, I invited Kristina and Susan to give a guest lecture in my class about the realities of sexual misconduct and assault cases. Given the confidential nature of campus sexual misconduct proceedings, many people have limited information about the kinds of sexual situations that come before these boards, let alone their options for a satisfactory resolution process (no matter what side of an allegation a person is on). Most people only hear about the most high-profile cases—the harrowing accounts of assaults by Harvey Weinstein, the conviction of Stanford swimmer Brock Turner, the discredited story of the gang rape at the University of Virginia. And I felt that my college students would benefit from hearing how some of the ways that people approach sex—and even view as norms—may actually be coercive or constitute assault.

After Kristina and Susan spoke to my students, I heard from a young woman in my class who was a survivor of sexual assault. She shared that, although she had initially felt wary of hearing from attorneys who hadn't just represented survivors but also those accused of sexual assault, she appreciated that Kristina and Susan were using what they had learned from their cases to educate others about sexual consent with the goal of preventing future sexual assaults. I also heard from men in my class who described having epiphanies where they realized they had previously done things during hookups that it hadn't occurred to them could make people feel frightened, overpowered, or coerced. Some described how hearing about the legal cases made them change how they approach sex—being more attentive to power dynamics, sexual communication, and consent. One shared that he didn't want to inadvertently harm someone by copying something he had seen in porn or learned to do from a friend.

Throughout this book, Kristina and Susan share some common kinds of sexual misconduct and sexual assault cases, with valuable insights that may shift some of your family's approaches to sensitive topics. In sharing these stories, none of us are trying to scare you. However, these are realities that must be considered, no matter how difficult the messages may be to hear and to discuss with one's child. It's just part of parenting today.

WHAT'S HERE AND WHAT'S NOT

As important as sexual consent is, this book addresses sexual consent as just one of many important conversations to have. Like others who have written on related topics (Christine Emba in *Rethinking Sex*, Lisa Damour in *Under Pressure*, Katherine Angel in *Tomorrow Sex Will Be Good Again*), I want to be clear: Consent is the bare minimum expectation when it comes to sex. It's important, but it's not sufficient for "good" sex that leaves people feeling valued or like their pleasure matters.

Yes, Your Kid is both an invitation and an update. It's an invitation to become closer with your child by being someone they can come to with questions, curiosities, and conundrums. To this end, you will find easy-to-follow ideas for conversations with your child—at every age and stage—related to bodies, puberty, boundaries, consent, sexual and reproductive health, technology, pornography, partnered sex, and more.

This book also provides an update to existing sex education materials, something that all parents need, whether they know it or not. There are many terrific sex education books for parents, but most were written in the "before times"—before sexting, before the COVID-19 pandemic, and before rough sex became the new norm. Given all that's changed in the world, parents need to learn what contemporary sex is like for young people. In writing this book, it also felt important to dedicate space to considering sexuality issues in the context of neurodiversity and, more specifically, autistic teens and young adults. In recent years, research and sexuality curricula have increasingly centered autistic voices. These insights are offered here to guide parents to support both neurodiverse and neurotypical kids.

Yes, Your Kid is not, however, a prescription. All children, and all families, are unique. Thus, I've included general recommendations for talks to have and approximately when to have these talks, making space for the flexibility to figure out what works for your family regarding your values, religion, and culture. It also feels important to note that this book is not "about" gender identity or approaches to gender affirmation. These are important topics, but they are also complex topics that deserve (and have) their own dedicated spaces in gender-focused books and websites. In *Yes, Your Kid*, the focus is on sexuality. However, where possible, I have shared research on how the sexuality topics addressed here are experienced by both cisgender and gender-diverse youth, as well as how parents can better support transgender and nonbinary kids on topics such as puberty, relationships, and sexual behavior.

In sections titled "What Do I Say?" I highlight some of the more common questions that children and parents ask as well as responses and perspectives for your consideration. In sections titled "Collective Wisdom," Kristina, Susan, and I highlight key messages to consider. Given my work as a sexuality researcher and educator, my day-to-day is often marked by young people asking questions about their bodies, romantic and sexual feelings, relationships, and breakups. Although students confide in me about their difficulties, too, I mostly get to hear about joy, love, curiosity, consensual sexual exploration, and questions along the lines of "Am I normal?" As attorneys, however, Kristina's and Susan's daily caseloads involve supporting young people and their parents as they navigate crisis situations related to sexual misconduct, sexual harassment, or sexual assault. Given our vastly different experiences, we don't always take the same perspective on a situation, and that's okay. In "Collective Wisdom," we find our areas of agreement and share them with you.

Having information about what sex is like for young people today and having tools to support these vital conversations can reduce your anxiety and boost your confidence as a parent. More than anything, I hope that reading this book helps you to feel like you and your family can learn to proactively talk about sex more comfortably and openly—not just through a single "talk" but through countless conversations. I hope that you feel better able to help your child avoid harmful situations but, should they occur, that you feel less alone and have some information on how to support them and what to do next. Romantic and sexual development are part of growing up. Being able to hear your child's questions, delight in their curiosity, and offer tools to think through complicated choices is a gift—both for them and for you. Let's begin.

1

"I Love That Question!"— Becoming an Askable Parent

Young people don't need their parents to be sex experts. However, they do benefit from having parents who are safe, loving people they can trust with their questions, worries, and big feelings about sex, bodies, and relationships. For simplicity, we'll call these "sex questions," even though they're so much more than that. Sex educators refer to this sense of openness as being an *askable parent*. Being askable doesn't mean always having the right answers. And sometimes there are no right answers. That's okay too. Being askable just means that your child sees you as someone who is open, approachable, caring, and welcomes their questions, curiosities, and observations.

HOW TO BECOME MORE ASKABLE

Becoming askable is a skill, and it's one we can learn, practice, and improve. What follows are some ideas about how to do that.

It Starts with Love

When I surveyed some college students on how parents could better support their teens when it came to sexuality issues, a first-year student said, "Just be an open ear. Sometimes you don't have to say anything. Just listen to your teen's experience and be a warm, comforting figure." Teens who have a close, caring, and supportive relationship with their parents tend to take fewer sexual risks and wait longer to have partnered sex.[3] Being supportive does not mean giving your child everything they want, shielding them from the consequences of their actions, or enabling bad behavior. Those responses hurt over time rather than help. Having a supportive relationship means that your child feels like you show them love and admiration. Young people who feel supported by their parents can be sure that their parents won't mock them or be overly critical of them—especially in front of their friends—such as by making fun of them for missing a goal or feeling afraid of the dark.

Showing affection is easy for some people and difficult for others. Even if your own family of origin was lacking in affection or support, you have a second chance with your own child. Showing affection might include patting them on their back, offering hugs or kisses, or saying "I love you." Showing admiration might involve saying:

- "I admire how much you care for your friends."
- "I'm impressed by how carefully you approach your schoolwork."
- "I've noticed how hard you work to improve at soccer and I'm proud of you."
- "Coming out to me and your mom took courage, which I admire in you."

Everyone needs to feel loved, cared for, and seen. Finding ways to show love and admiration are important parts of a supportive parent-child relationship.

Encourage Curiosity

Curiosity about romantic relationships and sexuality is developmentally normal, including for children and teens. Whether a child's parents are still together or apart, they often enjoy hearing origin stories about how their parents met, fell in love, and came to have children. And that curiosity can be a natural lead-in to important conversations about having children, finding a mate, nurturing a relationship, and what makes a relationship healthy or troubling. Unfortunately, children are sometimes shamed for this natural curiosity when they ask about sex.

In other contexts, parents often reward their child's curiosity by praising them for asking questions. When a child asks how long bears hibernate, a parent might say, "Great question!" and then either answer the question or look up the answer and learn together. Supportive responses teach young people that curiosity and learning are valued. Yet, for many parents, sex questions feel different, embarrassing, or stressful.

If you feel unprepared to respond to sexuality-related questions, you're not alone. I regularly hear from people who are facing challenging sex-related conversations with their child and want advice. "What do I say?" they ask. Or, "I thought I had a few more years before this would come up." Fortunately, with a little practice, you can become more calm, confident, and askable—no matter the question.

Even if you already feel open and approachable, be sure to broadcast this. When your child asks a question, respond with appreciation, encouragement, and shared curiosity. If their question feels distressing, take some breaths and find your center. Try to look calm, collected, and glad for their question; a warm smile helps. Say, "Great question!" or "I'm glad you asked that." Encourage them to share their ideas by asking, "What do you think?" or "What's your best guess?" Science-minded kids might have fun being asked, "What's your hypothesis?" In doing so, parents can engage them in the process of learning rather than always positioning themselves as experts who hold all the answers.

Asking what your child thinks also buys you time to breathe and collect your thoughts. It helps to follow up a "Good question!" by asking, "What have you heard about that?" This may give some context as to where the question came from: friends, cousins, television, the internet, or overheard on the school bus, for example. Having this information will help you understand what happened (Was it a developmentally appropriate situation? Did content filters fail? Might they have been abused?) as well as next steps you may need to take (answer the question and move on, fix content filters, or seek professional support).

If you don't know the answer, offer to learn more and circle back. This encourages your child's curiosity and shows that you take their questions seriously. With younger children, looking up information on your own may be preferable to searching the internet together as searches involving sex-related terms may bring you to websites with adult content. Say: "I'm going to search this privately first because the internet has some pictures and information that are only for grown-ups." That gives you time to find, sift through, and then share age-appropriate information or videos from which you both can learn. With teenagers, it can help to search the internet together—assuming you have filters or content settings applied to screen out adult content such as pornography. Searching with your child models how to find information, decide which websites are trustworthy, and critically evaluate what you learn.

Encouraging Responses to Kids' Questions

- "I'm glad you asked that. What have you heard?"
- "Great question! What are your thoughts?"
- "I love that you asked that question!"
- "Isn't that interesting to think about? Here's what I've heard."
- "What a neat thing you're wondering about! What's your hypothesis?"

Another option is to respond with "say more" or "tell me more about that." These are simple, easy, and nonjudgmental, an open invitation to hear what's on your child's mind.

Be Present

From puberty through adulthood, young people experience many milestones. Going with your child to purchase period products or showing them how to shave can lead to conversation as well as foster intimacy and trust. In contrast, avoiding any mention of these changes can create distance, unless a child shares that they'd prefer to manage something on their own. Respecting their privacy is important too.

Even if you don't fully understand what your child is going through, being a source of support rather than conflict means so much. Some of my students share that they counted the days to arriving on campus, not just because college felt like an exciting next stage of life for them, but because they wanted to get on birth control, get on PrEP (an HIV-prevention medication discussed in Chapter 3), or stop hiding their condom stash. These students' stories stand in stark contrast to students who felt, even in high school, that they could go to their parents for information or support, talk openly with them about their dating lives, count on them for healthcare needs (like birth control or hormones), and not have to hide who they are. When a child feels they need to hide something important from a parent, it's often because they're worried their parent won't love them for who they are. Even when you disagree with your child's choices, emphasize that you love them.

Stick to What They Ask

Kids want an answer—not a monologue. Stick to short, simple, and straightforward responses that use age-appropriate words and concepts. This provides the information they asked for while keeping them from feeling overwhelmed or bored by a lengthy response. If a child wants more information, they will usually ask follow-up questions. Let them lead the way.

Let's consider some examples. When young children ask how babies are made, it's often enough to say that some bodies make sperm and other bodies make eggs and, when the sperm and egg meet and join together, they may find a place in the uterus to grow into a baby. Some children might ask how the sperm and egg find one another, in which case you might say, "Most of the time, the sperm swim into the vagina, travel into the uterus and fallopian tubes, and then find the egg." Having simple, fact-based conversations is easier when a family uses body part terms such as *vulva*, *vagina*, *penis*, *scrotum*, and *uterus*; it's also helpful for neurodiverse kids when adults use clear terms like these rather than euphemisms like *balls* or *wee-wee*.

Older children might ask how sperm leave the body to find an egg. You can say that sperm leave through an opening at the end of the penis, and that this is the same opening that lets out pee. A child who has this foundational knowledge may one day grow curious and ask how the sperm leave the penis and get to the egg; this might lead you to share information with them about vaginal intercourse. Some parents may describe intercourse but invite curiosity by saying that vaginal intercourse is "the most common way that babies are made, but there are other ways too." Some kids will leave it at that; others will have their interest piqued by the "other ways," which may prompt questions about other forms of conception. This opens the door for conversations about donor-conceived pregnancies, surrogacy, adoption, and the various ways that families grow—especially important if one of these applies to your family.

Some children are ready and interested to hear about the various ways that babies are made at young ages, whereas others don't ask these questions until they are older. Most children ask for just one or two pieces of information at a time; they don't usually want the entire story the first time they ask. Also, it's common for children, as with adults, to retain only bits and pieces of what they're told, so don't be surprised if you find yourself answering the same questions at different ages.

When to Say More

A friend's six-year-old daughter, who had previously learned about sperm, eggs, and intercourse through a series of questions, one day posed a new question for her mom: "What do people do if they want to put their penis and vagina together, but don't want to get pregnant?" Keeping it short and simple, her mom said, "Great question!" and described birth control in age-appropriate terms ("medicines that people can take to keep their body from becoming pregnant").

For this kindergartener, that answer was sufficient. But if a teenager asked that same question, the stakes would likely feel—and be—higher. A parent might want to provide more details about birth control, including letting their teen know about trustworthy websites that provide detailed information about birth control methods. They might also ask their teen what they've heard about preventing pregnancy, what other questions they have about sex or pregnancy, whether they are thinking about becoming sexually active, and if they would like to make an appointment with a healthcare provider to discuss birth control. When my college students ask questions about birth control, they almost always tell me that they are already sexually active and wanting to choose a more effective method than whatever they are using (often condoms, withdrawal, or wishful thinking). Most say they haven't yet told their parents that they are sexually active.

When it's not clear whether there are bigger issues behind a question, look for a gentle way into your child's thoughts, as understanding the feelings or concerns behind the question can be helpful. Try asking: "What else are you wondering or worrying about?" A younger child asking how babies are made might just be curious about this basic fact of life, or they might be wondering if their parents are planning to have any more children and, if so, what that would mean for them. Similarly, a teenager asking about birth control might simply be curious, or they could be sexually active and wondering how to protect themself and their partner. A tween asking if they can join a GSA (gender and sexuality alliance) might just be asking for permission to join, or alternatively, they might be trying to gauge their parent's reaction to determine if they're a safe person to talk with about their attractions. Someone once told me that their fourteen-year-old asked what a hymen is and if it's normal to bleed when people first have sex. At the time, the daughter said she was "just curious," but days later she shared that she'd recently had intercourse for the first time, much to her parents' surprise.

Parent-child conversations are part art and part science. To some extent, you've got to trust your gut and what you know about your child. If they need to know something important beyond the questions they've asked, share it anyway. If a child asks what a blow job is, although you might start with "I'm glad you came to me with that question; what have you heard?" and (depending on their age) explain that it refers to when a person puts their mouth on someone else's penis, and is not something that kids should do, you probably wouldn't stop there. You would likely want to gently ask other questions, such as where they heard the term or what they've heard other people say about it. Tone is important here: Try to stay calm rather than accusatory. I often get questions from parents whose child has asked them what it means to "eat private parts" or "lick a vagina." Sometimes the child asking this question is in middle school, but increasingly these questions are relayed by parents of five- to ten-year-olds.

Start by calmly asking where they heard the term. In my professional experience, it's often the case that a child has heard older cousins or kids at school use these terms without any context—as just silly things they are saying without knowing what they mean. Other times these questions come about because a child has stumbled upon pornography and doesn't understand what they've seen. When they've seen pornography, more detailed conversations are warranted, and it's a reminder to check the filters on home and school computers and devices. And when there's a sense that someone has asked a child to do something sexual (or has harmed them), direct intervention and professional support are needed to protect the child and to address the other person's behavior.

For tweens and teens asking about oral sex, the question could just reflect general curiosity, but there's a good chance they or their friends have seen pornography too. Also, they may be thinking about becoming sexually active, already be sexually active, or facing sexual pressure from a peer at school or online. If so, take stock of the conversations you haven't had yet, as well as conversations that are worth repeating—for instance, concerning healthy relationships, consent, care, and boundaries—and emphasize that there is no rush to have any kind of sex. They need to know that sexually transmitted infections (STIs) can be passed through oral sex, and not just through vaginal or anal intercourse. And conversations about dealing with sexual pressure and coercion—and not being someone who pressures or coerces others—are critical too. (Don't worry; we'll cover each of these in the coming chapters.)

WHY WE TALK ABOUT SEX

Despite good intentions to talk with their teen or young adult about sex, many parents find it difficult to say much more than "don't have sex," "don't get pregnant" (or "don't get somebody pregnant"), "use a condom," or "wait until you're married." Some say nothing at all, hoping that their spouse or co-parent, or their child's school, will take on the sex talks. Yet, saying "don't have sex"—and little else—may send the message that sex is inherently bad or that you won't understand, love, or accept them if they make sexual choices that differ from your values. If your child feels sex is something they aren't even supposed to talk about, they will be less likely to ask questions and less likely to see you as a safe, trusted source for support.

It's more helpful to share about what sex is like in real life, which means describing both its joys and difficulties, as well as how people can protect themselves from harm. Leaving sex education to statements like "don't have sex" also ignores the reality that most teenagers have oral, vaginal, and/or anal sex with their peers. In the US, nearly 40 percent of high school students have had intercourse (an imprecise term that most young people probably take to mean vaginal intercourse), and most teens have had oral sex.[4] Among high school seniors, about 57 percent have had intercourse. Fewer teens have had anal sex, but some have (less than 5 percent, with higher rates among gay and bisexual boys as well as gender-diverse teens).[5]

Sex talks that can be summarized as "don't do it" just shut down conversation. Yet young people need to learn to talk about sex. In one study, college students who used nonverbal consent when having their first sexual intercourse (i.e., who consented to sex but didn't talk about it first) were less likely to use condoms or other forms of birth control when they had sex as compared to those who used verbal consent.[6] Learning to talk about sex has other benefits, too. My college students often say that, as they gain more experience talking about sex throughout our semester together, they begin to:

- Talk more comfortably with their parents about sex and relationships, leading them to feel closer with their parents and develop a better understanding of their family's values;
- Realize that it's okay to not be interested in sex, even if it seems like everyone around them is sexually active;
- Communicate more openly with their sexual partners, including discussing the kinds of sex they do or do not want to try, asking partners to stop something they don't like or that hurts, and asserting their boundaries;
- Learn how to create fun, pleasurable, respectful, and loving intimate relationships;
- Feel more comfortable disclosing their sexual orientation to a healthcare provider as well as seeking healthcare for their sexual health needs, including birth control, sexually transmitted infection (STI) testing, and help for painful sex.

Age-appropriate, fact-based, and compassionate sexuality education is good for families, relationships, communities, and individuals' sexual health. For college students, taking a human sexuality course not only helps improve partner communication, sexual pleasure, orgasm experiences, and comfort with sexuality topics, it also decreases students' feelings of needing to be secretive about sex, decreases homophobia, and reduces students' acceptance of acquaintance rape.[7] As for the idea that being taught about sex leads more young people to have sex, the research is clear that that's not the case either for teenagers or college students.[8] For students who want to wait to have sex until they are married (as some of my students plan to do and which I respect), taking a human sexuality course prepares them well in advance. They describe leaving class feeling optimistic about being able to one day create a mutually pleasurable and respectful sex life with their spouse. Students also share that they feel less anxious and more confident as a result of having learned about sex, pleasure, communication, and health. And for students who are not interested in having sex (whether right now or ever), they often develop new ways to communicate their feelings to friends and family, which can help them feel less anxious and more understood. Yet, some college students indicate that they're afraid to register for such a course, sharing that they worry their parents will judge or shame them. If your child is enrolled in college, encourage them to sign up for a sexuality-related course; these can often be found in departments related to health education, human development and family studies, sociology, or psychology.

HOW TO SHARE SEXUALITY INFORMATION

Now that we've talked through how to become a more askable parent, let's look at specific strategies for identifying what kinds of information or support your child may need as well as effective ways to initiate sexuality conversations. Try on what works for you and leave what doesn't. You've got this!

Listen Closely

Every child has their own pattern when it comes to opening up—rhythms around when they are more likely to talk freely. Some are late-night talkers, sharing stories about their friends or school day before drifting off to sleep. Others are chatty in the morning, asking big questions about life between bites of breakfast. Sometimes, it's less about the time of day than the conditions—opening up to a parent only when they have one-on-one time. When possible, spend time with your child when it aligns with their rhythms, knowing they're more likely to confide in you during these times.

Also, listen for moments when your child is sharing with friends or siblings. When your child has friends over and they're hanging out nearby while you're cooking dinner, keep your ears open. There may be a natural opportunity to interject or perhaps you will overhear something that gives you an idea for a later conversation. Some things you overhear might be lighthearted, such as joking about something funny that happened during their school's sex education class. Others may be more difficult, such as comments about a classmate who your child or their friends consider "slutty" or who has a high "body count" (a term used to refer to the number of sexual partners someone has had). This would be an ideal time to step in and challenge them on such comments, just as if you would if the comments were racist or ableist.

Sexual Identity Terms

Although some of these terms have been in use for decades, others may be new to you. Here are some I use throughout the book:

Asexual (ace): Someone who feels little to no sexual attraction to others or else feels some attraction to others but no need to act on those feelings.

Bisexual (bi or bi+): Attracted to people of more than one gender. A bi+ person may be attracted to other genders in equal amounts or in different amounts—such as mostly into women but a little into men or nonbinary people. Being bisexual has nothing to do with whether a person's relationships are open or monogamous.

Demisexual: Feeling sexually attracted to someone only after developing an emotional bond with them. Someone who is demisexual may also identify as gay, lesbian, straight, bisexual, or another sexual orientation.

Gay: A person who is attracted to people of their same gender.

Heterosexual: Sometimes referred to as "straight," this refers to women who are attracted to men and men who are attracted to women.

Lesbian: Usually refers to a woman who is primarily attracted to other women, though some women who are attracted to nonbinary people may identify as lesbians, too.

LGBTQ+: An acronym that refers to lesbian, gay, bisexual, transgender, queer, questioning, and other sexual and gender minorities within the community. Variations include LGBTQA+ ("A" for asexual) and LGBTQIA+ ("I" for intersex).

Pansexual (pan): Someone who is attracted to others regardless of their gender.

To learn more sexual orientation terms, check out glossaries from the It Gets Better Project or PFLAG (see **Resources**). And if you have a question about what your child's identity means for them, ask—just make sure the question is coming from a place of respect.

The goal isn't to eavesdrop; everyone deserves their privacy. But being intentional about listening lets you learn more about your child and the kinds of information or support that may benefit them.

DESCRIBE RATHER THAN JUDGE

Whether you're talking with your child about sex or other topics, consider describing—sticking to facts or what you observe—rather than offering judgments. If your child asks what condoms are, a judgment-based response (and, by the way, an inaccurate one) might be: "They're an unreliable form of birth control. Please don't ever be so foolish as to use condoms; that's asking for trouble." In contrast, a descriptive response might be: "Condoms are made from different kinds of thin material. The kind of condom most people use goes over the penis, but some other condoms can be used inside the vagina. People use condoms to reduce the risk of pregnancy and STIs."

When we're constantly expressing judgment of people, decisions, bodies, clothes, jobs, and so on (and we all do this sometimes), our kids may feel like they need to monitor our reactions to figure out where they fit and how to stay loved and accepted. It's difficult for a child to come to their parent with sensitive questions and conundrums if they fear being judged; it's easier to connect with a parent who they can just talk to.

DELIBERATE DISCUSSIONS

This approach may be the closest to "The Talk" many of us imagine occurring between parents and their children. Although sex education is an ongoing conversation, sometimes something occurs that will prompt a specific talk. For example, if you find condoms in your teen's room or porn sites in their web browser history, you may decide it's time for a chat. If having a specific sex talk is not an emergency (and it rarely is), it can help to first:

- Take time to cool down, especially if you're feeling shocked, scared, or triggered.
- Look for the positives. After all, if you found birth control pills in your teen's backpack, at least they are trying to be safe.
- Talk with your spouse, co-parent, or best friend.
- Prepare yourself. If you want to learn about a certain topic (STIs, birth control methods, school policies, what's typical for your child's age), take the time to do so. If it would help to role-play a conversation with a friend or co-parent, do that.
- Ask yourself questions like "What do I want my child to know?" and "How do I want them to feel?" and "What values do I want to share with them?"

When you do sit down together, start with love and support. Say something like, "Because I love you and want to give you the best guidance I can as a parent, I have something I want to talk with you about, even though this feels awkward for me and perhaps for you too." This lets your child know that you love them, that you are there to offer guidance (not a firm directive—unless that is needed, such as if they are doing something harmful or illegal), and that you value openness.

Then you talk together, with a goal of having a conversation rather than delivering a monologue. Try to embrace curiosity rather than place blame, shame, or make assumptions. "I'm curious why you have condoms" feels different than "I can't believe you have condoms and that you hid them from me!" Curiosity will help you to keep an open mind; besides, your child's answers may surprise you.

Teachable Moments

Streaming services and personal computer devices (like tablets) have made it common for family members to watch what they want to watch and to have fewer shows in common. While this has its upsides, there are drawbacks too. If you're watching different shows than your child, then you're missing out on chances to discuss what characters are doing and what you each think about their choices. Try to create some overlap in your media viewing. A friend and her high-school-aged stepdaughter created a tradition where they watch a classic movie from the 1980s or 1990s on weekends that they're together. Many of the films present natural teachable moments; for example, *Sixteen Candles* inspired a conversation about consent, and *There's Something About Mary* prompted frank talk about masturbation.

Some parents agree to let their teen join certain social media platforms (Instagram, TikTok) but only on the condition that the parent joins too, and that they are one another's friends or contacts on the platform. While the mere act of being connected online cannot prevent bad things from happening, it is a middle ground between oversight and total ignorance that works for some parents as they come to terms with their teens' path toward adulthood. Using this strategy helped one friend notice a TikTok trend that concerned her (it involved young women simulating a sex act on boys) and sparked a conversation between her and her eighth grader.

Whether it's social media or watching a TV show together, having common ground can inspire conversations and hopefully be a way to have fun together too. Looking for a show that does double duty by providing sex education and/or inclusive representation of young people's relationships and sexuality? Depending on your teenager's age, consider *Sex Education*, *Atypical*, *Heartstopper*, *Never Have I Ever*, *Big Mouth*, or *The Sex Lives of College Girls*.

Make Books Available

Many parents give their child age-appropriate books about bodies and sexuality. We're not (just) talking about Judy Blume books, but nonfiction books written for kids your child's age that delve into genital anatomy, reproduction, puberty, safer sex, sexual and gender identity, and/or sexual pleasure. These are books that kids can keep in their room and browse at their leisure. You might even leave sticky notes inside the book, pointing out sections you feel are important to read. If you have a shared collection of e-books or audiobooks, download age-appropriate books and let your child know that these have been added to your family library. You can also leave sex education books lying around the house to facilitate access to a trustworthy source when a question arises. A friend I grew up with described how, as a high school student, he had learned about sex by reading his parents' copy of the classic book *The Joy of Sex*.

Having valuable resources at home in book form can make a huge difference. For one, if a child has engaging, informative sex education books, they may be less likely to feel compelled to search the internet or seek out pornography to learn about sex. And even if they do turn to these sources, at least their viewing will be balanced out by a broader media diet that includes good-quality sex education books. Sharing trustworthy, nonjudgmental books with your child can also signal that you see who they are and who they're on the path to becoming, and that you're there to support their growth. As one in six teenagers identifies as other than heterosexual (gay, lesbian, bisexual, pansexual, asexual, queer, etc.), make sure that the books you choose are LGBTQ+ inclusive (see **Resources**). And if you live in a community affected by school book bans (many of which target books with LGBTQ+ characters), ask your child if there are any books they'd like to be able to read, but haven't yet been able to access. Buying these books, or checking them out from the local library, can expand their world and show your support.

Even if you share books with your child, it's still wise to talk together about sex. Say that you are giving these books to your child because you love them and because your family values openness and bodily autonomy. A person can't be fully in charge of their own body if they don't have sufficient information about their body, how it works, and how to keep themselves safe. Then consider adding, "When you have questions about sexuality, I hope you will come to me or, if you're not coming to me, I'd feel more comfortable with you going to (name other trusted adults) or reading this book rather than searching the internet." If your child is a teenager and/or already knows what pornography is, caution against trying to learn about sex from watching pornography and why. The idea is to send the message that you see the book as just one part of your child's sex education—not that you are using a book to avoid talking with them.

Five Minutes a Week

Some parents tell their teen that talking and learning about sex and relationships is so fundamental that they are going to do it often. They may say, "While I understand that these talks can be awkward, they're important, so once each week I'm going to set a timer for five minutes, and we're going to talk about sex, love, or relationships. When the timer is up, we can stop talking or keep talking—it'll be up to you." Some parents find that, after a few five-minute sex talks, their teen begins coming to them with more questions and initiating longer conversations. Moreover, studies show that teens who have more frequent, even repetitive, sex talks with their parents feel closer to their parents, feel like they have a more open relationship with their parents, and feel better able to communicate with their parents not just about sex but overall.[9]

To start, read a page from an age-appropriate sex education book or watch sex education videos together (see **Resources**). Or open by asking what kinds of questions they have or by talking through a scene from a television show that you saw together and that's been on your mind. You can also flip the conversation around and ask your teen about something you've been curious about and that they seem to be knowledgeable about, such as a gender or sexual orientation term that is new to you or why a certain song or video is controversial.

"I Learned Something New"

It can be difficult to know how to begin a conversation about sex. Leading with "I learned something new" is a strategy that works for some parents. A colleague told me about the time he said to his older teen, "I heard that there's porn on Twitter—did you know that?" His son did in fact know that and had previously come across porn on Twitter, and this began a conversation about what they each thought, and how such images were readily accessible. Another friend who is an avid reader of historical nonfiction likes to share with her family what she learns. What does historical nonfiction have to do with what sex is like for young people today? As it turns out, quite a lot. My friend has learned about the history of birth control laws and the diverse ways people have expressed their gender through time and around the world, as well as pivotal moments related to sex and relationships like the Stonewall uprising and *Loving v. Virginia*. She reads, learns, and starts conversations with her family.

Some parents may worry that saying they've just learned A, B, or C will make them seem uncool or out of touch. Although that could happen, letting go of the need to seem cool has its rewards—including educating your teen and creating more open conversations. Admitting you've learned something new also demonstrates that no one has all the answers and that it helps to stay curious. Besides, teenagers already tend to think their parents are out of touch; what have you got to lose?

Sex Ed in the Car

Some parents like to broach the topic of sex when their child is a captive audience, such as while driving to or from school, sports, dance class, or other activities. My college students often write about how, back when they were in middle school or high school, their parent would use this time to talk with them about sex. Sometimes they jokingly describe feeling "trapped," but also note a big upside: they didn't have to make eye contact during these awkward sex talks. Not only do my students remember these conversations, but they generally say that they're grateful to their parent for having put in the effort.

Unfortunately, thanks to smartphones and other devices, car rides may not offer as much of a captive audience situation as they used to, when car rides were just a parent, a kid, and a car radio. Try asking your child to set aside their phone while you're in the car together to help make dedicated space for conversation.

Let Them Listen In

No matter how askable you are, it's common for children to avoid talking with their parents about sexual topics. A friend of mine devised a brilliant solution for her family. She had noticed that whenever she and her husband tried to catch up with one another about their day, their teenager would listen in, interrupting them with questions like "What happened?" or "Who said that?" My friend realized that even though their daughter didn't want to sit down with them for sex talks, she seemed drawn to her parents' private conversations. Seizing on that curiosity, my friend and her husband began to intentionally create conversations about sexuality topics ("I read today that chlamydia rates are rising"), fully aware that their daughter would listen more closely if she had the sense that these were "grown-up conversations." As expected, the daughter started listening in and asking questions, which resulted in robust family conversations about sex and relationships.

To try this out, take something you've learned from reading this book or have seen in the news and, within earshot of your child, chat about it at home with your spouse or partner, or over the phone with a friend. The conversations you let your child listen in on can be based on fact or focused on feelings and values. For example, letting them overhear you talk with your partner or friend about the importance of love and support for LGBTQ+ youth may broadcast to your kid that you are an askable and accepting parent. Remember: your child is likely listening in no matter what; this is a chance to be more intentional about what you're saying.

Advocate for School-Based Sexual Health Education

Studies spanning several decades have found broad public support for comprehensive school-based sexuality education. Most parents—regardless of political party—support middle school and high school sex education on abstinence, birth control, sexual orientation, healthy relationships, STIs, and puberty.[10] It's not enough for your own child to be educated about sex if their present or future partners have had dismal sex education. And while most parents want to play an active role in their child's sexuality education, we can all use some help. Mothers, especially, tend to take on the extra work of being their child's primary sex educator[11] (on top of other household and parenting tasks disproportionately done by women). School-based sexuality education supports kids, takes pressure off parents, and creates more equitable experiences across the board. Consider advocating for comprehensive sexuality education in your state or local school district, which is where many curricular decisions are made (see SIECUS.org).

WE ALL MAKE MISTAKES

When talking with your child about sex, be prepared to make mistakes. Your child may ask you something about sex, or you may overhear something that you react to in a way you wish you hadn't. You may withdraw, get mad, or say, "Why would you even ask such a thing?" We have all had the experience of not living up to our ideals. Fortunately, we can start over. Try saying, "That conversation didn't go as I had hoped" or "I'm sorry I snapped at you. You asked such a good question, and I love how open you were with me. Can we try again?" Not only does this help you have the conversation you want, and with a more supportive tone, but it also models for your child how to repair a missed moment of connection.

Collective Wisdom

Now that we have the "how" part down, the next chapter shares specific topics for discussion such as body parts, masturbation, consent, and healthy relationships. As you start these conversations, keep in mind: ·

1. **You can do this!** If you've found yourself saying, "I should talk with my child about (fill in the blank)," this is an opportunity to make a plan for a conversation, and change your "I should" to an "I will."

2. **Start with love.** A loving, supportive relationship with your child gives them someone to bring questions to; it also gives them a trusted person to turn to if or when something difficult happens to them. If your child groans and gives you the "Stop being weird!" treatment when you try to connect, say, "I understand it can feel weird, but I love you and this information is important to your health and future relationships, so I want to be sure I share it with you."

3. **Let them see you sweat.** Having an awkward conversation shows your child that it can be done. It feels difficult at first, we learn we can do it, and then we grow more confident as a result. That's a wonderful thing for your child to witness.

4. **Don't feel pressured to answer personal questions.** It's healthy to draw
    boundaries as to what you are and are not comfortable sharing with your
    child, just as they will understandably draw boundaries with you. If they ask
    a question that feels too personal, say, "I understand your curiosity, but that's
    private." You might be comfortable sharing certain things (such as how you
    decided on a form of birth control or traits that were important to you in a
    partner) but feel that other things are off-limits. Setting healthy boundaries is
    good for everyone.

2

The Talk: It's Never Too Early (or Late) to Start

Rather than a single talk, parents will ideally have hundreds of age-appropriate talks with their child about bodies, relationships, love, attraction, conception, sexual orientation, and partnered sex. Potty training offers frequent opportunities to name body parts ("next, wipe your vulva"). A child whose family is expecting a baby may be curious about how babies are made, birth, or the adoption process. Young people who have a disability, or a family member with a disability, might be more likely to ask questions about how disabled people make love or give birth. And puberty, periods, and early experiences with ejaculating (nocturnal emissions, also called "wet dreams") bring up their own anxieties and questions.

In this chapter, you will find a discussion of body and sexuality topics that commonly come up in families, or that parents might want to bring up at some point, as well as ideas for how to approach these topics. Because kids and families vary, as do their needs, there's no simple chart of which talks to have at which ages. Also, this chapter does not reflect every single topic you should or may want to discuss, as children are full of surprises with the questions they ask and the information they crave. I've intentionally included ideas for talks from early childhood through adolescence and young adulthood. Even if you think you're past a certain stage with your own child, please read the entire chapter. You never know if they will one day ask questions about topics that you thought were long ago resolved. Kids (like adults) forget things and ask again; they also return to a topic for additional detail and complexity as they understand more or hear conflicting or confusing information from peers.

Foundational Topics

Body Basics
- Naming Body Parts
- How Bodies Work
- Puberty and Periods

Body Sovereignty
- Greetings
- Boundaries
- Consent
- Freely Given Affection
- Ethical Persistence
- Inappropriate Touch

Relationships
- Healthy (and Unhealthy) Relationships

- "Catching Feelings"
- Power and Control
- Breakups and Rejection

Sexual Exploration
- Masturbation
- Vibrators and Sex Toys
- Sexual Pleasure
- Orgasm
- Sexual Orientation
- Partnered Sex
- Healthy Sexuality

In later chapters, I focus in detailed ways on sexuality topics that have experienced a sea change in recent years and so need more space. These include sexual consent, birth control, STIs and HIV, sex and technology, pornography, and rough sex, as well as special considerations for sexuality education for autistic kids. In this chapter, the focus is on a range of foundational topics, from puberty to healthy relationships. How you approach these conversations will be shaped by your family's values, culture, religion, and your child's questions, but the topics themselves are essential to supporting a lifetime of conversations between you and your child.

BODY BASICS

Everyone deserves to have information about their bodies, including how their bodies work and what changes to expect with puberty. This group of topics are the building blocks for conversations about valuing and respecting one's own body.

Naming Body Parts

From day one, it's important to give children language for talking about their bodies, including their genitals. I tend to favor terms such as *vulva*, *vagina*, *penis*, and *scrotum*. Some people call these the "correct terms," though I appreciate how sexuality educator Cory Silverberg, in their book *You Know, Sex*, honors the words that people feel are right for them (rather than asserting what is "correct"). Whatever terms your family uses at home, it's still helpful for children to be familiar with those that are commonly used by doctors and nurses; this makes healthcare appointments easier to understand. Also, words like *vulva* and *penis* are more straightforward, and less confusing, than euphemisms such as *down there* or *wee-wee*.

During diaper changes, you can say out loud: "After I clean your vulva, I'll get you a dry diaper." Although a newborn doesn't yet understand words, saying them anyway gives parents practice at becoming comfortable saying words like *vulva* and *penis* out loud. By the time older infants begin to learn words, these will be among them; infants and young toddlers are already learning language, even if there are few words they can form on their own yet. Not only does naming body parts help with potty training, but knowing and using widely understood words for body parts may make children less likely targets for child sexual abuse.[12] In the unfortunate event that a child is abused, having language to describe what happened can support them in talking with their parents, social workers, and/or police interviewers.[13] As a college professor, I have had several students tell me that taking my course and practicing saying body- and sexuality-related words out loud during class discussions helped them feel able to tell their healthcare provider that they had been sexually abused or assaulted. Words matter; sometimes they are a lifeline.

As lawyers handing sexual misconduct cases, Kristina and Susan talk with college students about sex nearly every day. Some students lack the language to describe what happened to them during an assault and need to be given diagrams to help them communicate where they were touched or penetrated. Others tell Kristina and Susan that these conversations are the first time they've used clinical words instead of slang (e.g., *breasts* instead of *titties*). And in my experience as a professor, every semester, a show of hands reveals that most students in my human sexuality course had never heard the word *vulva* prior to the first day of class, even though more than half of the students have one.

If your child is transgender or nonbinary, they may have preferred terms for their genitals (*front hole* instead of *vagina* and *T-dick* or *cock* instead of *clitoris*, for some trans men; *junk* or *girldick* instead of *penis*, for some trans women). Learning their preferred terms can improve your conversations with them about puberty or sexuality. In research interviews with study participants, I often say "I want to use words that feel right to you, and respectful of you, so can you please tell me what words you'd like me to use for your genital parts?" Participants usually thank me for asking and then share the words they prefer. My gender-diverse students often say that, as long as their family and friends ask them questions from places of care and respect, they're open to sharing their feelings and perspectives, so don't be afraid to ask about their preferred terms. And if they don't want to share those details, that's fine too. Say, "I respect your privacy; you can come and talk with me anytime you want."

How Bodies Work

Beyond naming body parts, make sure to share what they do—whether those functions seem mundane, awe-inspiring, or funny. Sharing how bodies work will help your child feel more informed and confident in conversations with their friends and future partners. No one wants to be the last kid in their class to learn how babies are made or what an orgasm is. Chapter 3 includes examples of how some parents talk with their children about the various ways people grow their families, but there are many needed talks to have aside from conception. When age-appropriate opportunities arise through reading books or answering questions, you might say that:

- Babies grow inside the uterus (with age, parents may introduce terms like *embryo* and *fetus* to describe different stages of development).
- Eggs are made and stored in the ovaries.
- Sperm are made and stored in the testes.
- Semen is a fluid that carries sperm in it and leaves the penis through a tube called the *urethra*. This same tube carries urine from the bladder.
- Erections happen when more blood flows into the penis than leaves the penis; during puberty, they happen in all sorts of situations and don't necessarily have anything to do with sexual thoughts.
- Sperm starts being made at puberty, which is often between ages ten and twelve, but may be earlier or later for some.
- The vagina is also called the *birth canal*, as most babies are birthed through it. The vagina stretches during delivery and then returns to its usual size. Babies can also be birthed through a surgery called a *C-section*, which is performed by a doctor.
- Menstruation usually begins between ages nine and fourteen (though earlier for some and later for others). The lining of the uterus breaks

down, releasing blood through the vagina. This is called *having a period*, and it usually happens for a few days each month. Pads, tampons, menstrual cups, and period underwear help people manage their bleeding.

- Periods are natural and nothing to be ashamed of. Although some people have some cramping, pain should not be so severe that it interferes with sports or school.
- On a vulva, the urethra (where pee comes out of) is just below the clitoris and above the vagina but is difficult to see because it's so small.
- The clitoris is packed with nerve endings and its only purpose is to feel things; it may feel good and sensitive to touch. (Many adult women say they learned this too late, so let teens know that clitoral stimulation makes it easier for many people to experience pleasure and orgasm.)
- The vagina is only a few inches long and ends at the cervix, meaning that a tampon (or condom) won't "get lost" into an abyss.
- Although the vagina is small, it expands during sexual arousal, which can make intercourse more comfortable.
- Vaginal lubrication also helps make penetration more comfortable and pleasurable; it builds up through spending time doing sexual things that people find arousing.

When it comes to vulvas, vaginas, and periods, tweens and teens are often relieved to hear that (1) it's safe to swim while menstruating, (2) period blood trickles out (rather than gushing like a faucet), and (3) vaginas don't smell bad or like fish (unless someone has an infection, which is why strong odors should be mentioned to one's healthcare provider). Also, it's common for labia (vaginal lips) to be asymmetrical—just as eyes, ears, and breasts are asymmetrical too.

As far as penis facts go, teenagers often have questions about size and its capacity to please (eventual) partners. Boys often get the message that they will need to "perform" well at sex and that big penises are better than small penises. Thus, they find it helpful to hear that: (1) the penis doesn't usually reach its full adult size until around age seventeen; (2) the average erect penis length is about five and a half inches (nowhere near pornographic norms); and (3) penis size has very little to do with whether sex is pleasurable for one's partner (but emotional intimacy does).

Puberty and Periods

Countless students have shared stories of panic arising during their pubertal years—usually because no one had told them about puberty before they experienced it firsthand. Knowing nothing about menstruation, some saw blood in their underwear and thought they were dying. Others worried they had hurt their body when they first ejaculated, as no one had ever mentioned masturbation, semen, or wet dreams. I've heard from many women who didn't understand why there were white stains and gooey stuff on their underwear, because no one had ever told them about vaginal discharge, which begins around puberty as estrogen levels increase. (Coincidentally, three of these young women finally learned that vaginal discharge is a normal part of having a vagina through watching an Amy Schumer skit, underscoring the value of having diverse voices represented in the media.) So please—do talk with your child about puberty, starting years before you expect it to begin. Puberty can feel frustrating because it happens on its own unpredictable schedule and is beyond one's control; having information can help young people feel more prepared.

Regarding periods, share that they mark a new phase of life (the reproductive years) and the beginning of ovulation (the release of eggs). The ovaries usually release one egg per month and, if there's no pregnancy, a period follows roughly two weeks later. That means that most people have a period each month, though periods are often irregular for the first year or two. Also, people bleed for different lengths of time—some for a few days, others for a week or longer. What a person calls their period (*period, monthly, flow*) is one of the few period-related things they have a say over, so honor your child's preferred language as well as how they wish to manage their periods, whether through tampons, pads, menstrual cups, or period underwear.

Also, say that while cramping is common, period pain should not be debilitating. Tell a healthcare provider if that's the case.

Trans and nonbinary teens who menstruate (not all do; even those with ovaries and a uterus may not, especially if they're using certain medications) may feel extra dysphoric around this time. The individual bathroom stalls in men's rooms often lack trash receptacles, and carrying used pads or tampons out of the stall to throw them away can be difficult to do without others noticing. Also, boxers aren't compatible with pads, which can complicate underwear options during menstruation. In offering support to your child around period-related issues, say, "I get that you may feel frustrated or dysphoric when you bleed, and there are likely things I don't understand about your experience, but I love you and I'm here for you if you want to tell me what you need or brainstorm how to make menstruation easier on you."

BODY SOVEREIGNTY

Body sovereignty refers to the idea that we are all in charge of our own bodies. This relates to what we eat, what we wear, and who we hug or kiss, as well as with whom we're sexual and when (if ever). Teaching your child that they are in charge of their own body is important. You can reinforce body sovereignty by giving your child the chance to make choices about their own body, something that's easy to do for low-stakes decisions (what to wear, whether they want to give hugs or high fives when they greet family). Also, reinforce their own body self-awareness and choices when possible. For example, if you encourage them to finish their dinner and they say they're full, say "Okay, you know your body best" and leave it at that.*

---

* If your child has or has had an eating disorder, this example may not apply; ask their healthcare provider how you can best support your child at mealtimes.

Greetings

Even before the #MeToo movement, there was increasing attention to the issue of greetings and farewells—specifically, the idea that hugs and kisses should be viewed as optional, not expected. Some people pushed back against this, suggesting that in some cultures or families there was no room for flexibility. Yet, people frequently adapt how they say hello and goodbye, such as when visiting other countries or during the COVID-19 pandemic, when people began waving from six feet apart (friendly yet distanced) or offering elbow bumps instead of handshakes or hugs. Respecting others' choice of greetings is important. There are many reasons someone may not want to hug or kiss hello. Some people don't want lipstick on their cheek. Others have sensory issues that make kisses painful, unexpected touch frightening, or bodily closeness uncomfortable.

Whatever the reason, if your child does not want to hug or kiss, they shouldn't have to. Encourage your child to offer high fives or waves instead. If someone says, "I'm a hugger!" and comes in close for a hug, they can accept the hug if they want one or else simply wave or offer a handshake. If your child wants to hug or kiss a peer, tell them to ask first and then kiss or hug only if the other person says yes. Or they can make room for options by asking, "High five, hug, or handshake?" If your teen works as a babysitter or camp counselor, talk with them about body boundaries when it comes to the children they're watching.

Some family members might get upset if your child says no to their hug or kiss. Share how the ability to say "no" and "stop" is important both for your child's comfort and their safety—and that the best place to practice that is among people with whom they feel close. Learning to respect other people's body boundaries will also help your child make and keep friends as a tween and teen.

Boundaries

From early ages, talk about family rules and boundaries around bathing, sleeping, using the bathroom, dressing, and media use. Name these boundaries and ask that they be respected. Boundaries will look different for different families, and they vary by culture. Boundaries also change as children grow older and no longer need help or supervision for bathing, bathroom, and dressing needs. All family members have rights to privacy in these personal areas of life. If a family member or friend is not honoring these rights, then as a parent you need to enforce the rules. You can model and communicate setting boundaries by:

- Being clear that your child can choose whether they want a hug or a kiss—even from a grandparent (as described earlier). Also, be clear that they should ask others before hugging or kissing them.
- Knocking (and waiting for permission) before entering someone's room or bathroom.
- Teaching a child that you will respect their "no" or "stop," and that other people should respect these words too. During tickle games or roughhousing, teach your child that if they say "no" or "stop," you will immediately stop.
- Letting family members know when you need space ("I'm going to take a nap; unless it is urgent, please give me my space and I'll come back when I'm done napping").
- Letting kids know, when they first start using family members' phones and cameras to take pictures, "Ask before taking a picture of someone" and "We only take pictures when people are wearing clothes." These comments lay the foundation for later talks about digital privacy and sexting.

Setting clear family rules about boundaries is important. Using words to communicate boundaries gives kids practice hearing about others' boundaries as well as experience communicating their own boundaries. Encourage your child to verbalize what they need—to use words rather than make you guess what they mean by a grunt, eye roll, or wordless retreat into their room. And while voicing boundaries is important, respecting those boundaries is the critical next step. If a child's boundaries are respected within their family and within their home, and their "no" and "stop" are heeded, then it will be easier for them to notice concerning behavior in others, such as people who disregard their no or make light of their boundaries.

Also, share that families are different in terms of their personal boundaries and rules. Just as some families have stricter curfews, some families are more relaxed about changing clothes or peeing in front of other family members, or posting pictures of their kids online. Children can learn differences but still understand that their family's rules guide their personal behavior.

Consent

When we disentangle consent from sex, we broaden opportunities to talk about the subject with kids of all ages. For many people, the word *permission* is more easily understood than *consent*. Use what fits best for your family. Teaching your child to ask if it's okay to borrow something sets the stage for more complex conversations later around boundary setting and, eventually, sexual consent.

There are many ways to address consent that have nothing to do with sex, such as:

- Setting a rule that family members ask before borrowing another family member's clothes.
- Asking before taking a picture of your child or others.
- Limiting posts about, and pictures of, your child on social media until they are old enough to decide for themselves.
- Pointing out consent violations. If your child tells you a story about how they and their friends drew pictures on a peer's face or removed some of their clothing after the peer feel asleep at a sleepover party (or passed out drunk at a college party), talk about how their peer was unable to give permission while they were asleep or passed out.

While this may seem to some like a harmless prank, waking up to realize what happened may make them feel embarrassed, ashamed, anxious, or violated.

As kids grow older, expand consent conversations to address sexual consent. Tell your child not to touch or grab other people's bodies or touch their hair without their permission. Many middle school and high school girls have had their butt or breasts grabbed, often in public as they're moving down the hallway to go to class. If your child is age ten or older, and it's been a while since you've talked about these topics, check in again, before the ages when these behaviors are known to escalate. Also, review school policies to understand how they define and address verbal and physical sexual harassment and make sure to talk with your child about how not to harass others (more on this in Chapter 5).

Freely Given Affection

Six-year-old Aspen, who was in a multi-age classroom, came home from school one day and told her mom that a younger classmate, who was four, had asked a teacher for help with their jacket's zipper. Aspen shared that the teacher, instead of immediately helping the child, said to the four-year-old, "Only if you hug me first." While this was likely meant as a playful comment, it sends the wrong message. It suggests that, to get help for a basic need (feeling warm on the playground on a wintry day), the child had to hug the teacher, whether they wanted to or not. It suggests that the teacher, rather than the child, is in charge of the child's body. That's not okay. Even at early ages, parents (and teachers) can model that affection should not be pressured, coerced, or insisted upon by others.

Sadly, sexual pressure and coercion are common. For teenagers and adults, one person may withhold something until the other person does something sexual for them. I've heard too many similar stories: the guy who wouldn't drive his date home unless they "at least" gave him a hand job; the young woman who refused to leave her ex's apartment unless he had sex with her "just one last time"; the college student whose restaurant manager wouldn't let her leave work early one night unless she flashed her breasts for him.

Young children will still have to do some things they may not want to for their health or safety, like hold hands while crossing a busy street, but kids should get to make most choices about their own body—including when to give and receive affection. For older children, you can share age-appropriate examples of feeling pressured or coerced. You may have your own memories of being nagged, guilted, or pressured into a hug, kiss, or sexual act. Sharing those memories, depending on a child's age and developmental stage, can underscore your point.

- A parent of a five-year-old might say, "When I was a kid, I had an uncle who would ask me to kiss him hello, but I didn't want to. And I want you to know that you never have to kiss or hug someone who you don't want to kiss or hug—even if it's someone in our family. Listen to your body. I trust you."
- A parent of a teenager might share, "When I was in high school, I went out with someone who treated me to dinner using their own money. But I was taken aback when they suggested I owed them oral sex, since they'd paid for my dinner. Although they then acted like it was just a joke, it still made me feel scared. I want you to know that you never owe anyone anything sexually, no matter how much money they spend on you, and even if they try to guilt you into it or tell you that you led them on. You get to decide what's right for your body. Further, no one owes you any kind of sex just because you buy them anything, either. They get to make choices about their own body too."

Emphasize that your child shouldn't take advantage of other people. Say that it is never okay to verbally or physically pressure people into hugs, kisses, or any kind of sex. Catchphrases like "your body belongs to you" and "they get to make their own choices about their body" should be repeated often.

Ethical Persistence

As you talk with your child about the importance of working hard and improving in school, sports, or hobbies, be clear that while persistence is admirable, they still need to respect other's people's bodies and their boundaries—especially in sexual situations. Some young people say that they've always been told to "try and try again," not to accept a no, or to work hard to turn someone's no into a yes. They may apply these same ideas to asking someone out or being sexual with them. Yet, people need to understand the difference between ignoring people's boundaries (not okay) and what writer Roxane Gay calls "ethical persistence,"[14] which involves learning to accept rejection and respecting other people's boundaries. At school, kids should not pester teachers to bump up their grade. At a party, if a friend says they don't want a beer, that choice should be respected; no one should try to wear them down until they agree to drink alcohol. And when it comes to sex, say, "If someone says no to a kiss or some kind of sex, or seems uninterested, move on. If they want to be sexual with you, they will let you know."

Inappropriate Touch

Most children explore their own bodies (including their genitals) by themselves as well as with siblings and/or peers, such as by playing doctor or showing one another their nude body parts. Pediatricians and child psychologists note how common and normative this play is among young children; it doesn't usually signal anything wrong or unusual. However, sometimes children experience situations that make them feel afraid or unsafe. Especially for young children, this can include nonconsensual interactions like having their underwear pulled down or their genitals touched by another child, even though they said no or tried to get away. It can also include feeling pressured to play games like "I'll show you mine if you show me yours." For older kids and teens, unwanted and nonconsensual touching of breasts and butts, as well as genital slapping or wet-towel thwacking between boys as part of locker room hazing, are all too common. And from college men, I've heard stories of fraternity hazing that was sexual in nature and felt humiliating.

If your child experiences nonconsensual touch, they may want to process the experience with you. Listen to them, validate their feelings, and help them to identify safe ways forward. This might include you, as the parent, speaking with a teacher or principal to create a safe school environment, which often includes closer supervision. If an experience crosses the line into abuse or something illegal, safe ways forward should include reaching out for professional advice and support.

You can offer love, reassurance, and a listening ear to your child and still find that their fears linger. It may take days or weeks (or longer) before your child stops talking about the incident. Chances are, your child will eventually work out the issue, especially if given the time, space, and support to do so. Validating your child's feelings can help ("I understand; that was wrong for Sam to grab your penis and I would feel mad too"). It can also help to focus on your child as a whole person, so that having been inappropriately touched doesn't define them. When the moment passes and you spot an opening, ask them about a painting they've been working on or the math test they had at school. This is not to dismiss your child's concerns; their worries are real and should be heard. But zooming out to the bigger picture of their lives can help so they don't feel trapped in their worry. And if your child needs more time to process, give them the time and attention. If you're unsure whether your child needs extra support, contact a therapist who works with kids your child's age. It's upsetting to see one's child feeling unsafe, and it may bring up feelings of times when you felt unsafe, or when those around you didn't offer enough protection. You may want to process your own feelings with a friend, co-parent, spouse, or your own therapist; by all means, care for yourself as you care for your child.

If your child has touched another child's body or genitals in a way the other child did not want or agree to, try to learn more about what happened. If they did something unusual for their age (such as a young child trying to simulate oral sex or intercourse) or in a way that worries you, the behavior deserves a closer look. Sometimes this happens because the child once walked in on their parents having sex and are reenacting what they saw; other times it reflects having stumbled upon pornography, which should prompt parents to check search filters, more closely monitor device use, and talk with their child about what they saw. The behavior may also signal that your child has been inappropriately touched by an older child or adult, which warrants professional support.

Even if the way your child touched a peer was in the typical range of behavior, if it was done without permission, do talk with your child about consent and boundaries, as well as family or school rules. You can say to a young child, "Even if another child says it's okay, your school has a rule against kissing one another, as well as rules against touching one another's vulva or penis, so please don't do that." For older kids and teens who have nonconsensually touched other kids' breasts or butts at school, such as in the hallway, have a talk about how unsafe that can feel. Talk about sexual harassment and assault and how serious they are, how violated they can make other people feel, and that they are against school policies.

Finally, many schools include age-appropriate books on consent for children as part of story time (for younger children) or on the classroom bookshelf (for older children). Ask how your child's school teaches about body boundaries and consent.

RELATIONSHIPS

Although it often seems like young people are most interested in learning about sex, they often want to learn about dating and relationships more than they let on. From day one, human beings are intimate creatures. Babies are soothed by skin-to-skin contact. One reason they cry is to signal that they want to be held. Those basic human needs, including what some call "skin hunger" (the need to be touched), never go away, and relationships are how we meet those needs. Here are some key messages to share on this vital topic.

Healthy (and Unhealthy) Relationships

At all ages, families can model, as well as discuss, healthy relationship characteristics. Humans have close relationships (family members, good friends, best friends, romantic partners) as well as less intimate ones (more distant family members, classmates, teachers, among others). Feeling close and connected to others, and like one belongs, matters. Helping your child learn to thrive in their friendships and relationships, resolve disagreements, and recognize both healthy and unhealthy patterns of behavior is a gift to their present and future selves.

Although most of us could create a long list of characteristics we value in a friend or partner, distilling the key features of a healthy relationship into a few essentials makes them easier to talk about with younger children. When I've asked young children what they like about being around their close friends, they've said:

- We have fun together.
- We laugh a lot.
- I feel good around them.
- They don't hurt me.
- They don't make fun of me.

Kids get it: they want to feel safe, good inside, and like they can be themselves. Talking with your child about these key features of healthy relationships—and repeating them throughout their childhood and adolescence—gives your child a framework for how to think about their friendships. As they grow older and start to date or develop crushes, they will hopefully keep asking themselves: *When I'm with this person, do I feel safe, good inside, and like I can be myself?*

In my own life, I remember becoming friends with someone new in middle school (we'll call her Nina, though that wasn't really her name). Nina seemed smart and funny but, as we spent time together, I saw that she could also be mean. One day, Nina spread a hurtful rumor about a boy in our class who kids often teased. The rumor wasn't a lie, but it was private information that she shouldn't have shared without our classmate's permission. I was standing there when Nina told a group of classmates his information, and I didn't know what to do or say. But I did know that I felt awful inside, and that I'd seen enough meanness to know I could no longer be her friend. This is a story I've shared with my own children because I want them to understand how important it is to examine one's own friendships and relationships and grow from difficult moments. I've shared similar stories with them about dating and how important it was for me to identify what I liked, as well as what I didn't like, about relationship partners.

Aside from the basics of feeling safe, good inside, and like one can be themselves, there are other aspects of healthy relationships that parents can talk about with their child, especially as the child grows older and capable of more complex conversations. For example, in healthy relationships, people:

- Support and encourage one another.
- Care how the other person is feeling, both in the moment and later on.
- Lift one another up ("you're so smart" and "you can do it!") rather than tear one another down ("you're a failure" or "you'll never get anywhere in life").
- Are happy when the other person has fun with their friends and family (in contrast, a "red flag" is when someone tries to keep their friend or partner from hanging out with others).
- Have healthy disagreements.
- Don't pressure or coerce each other into doing things they don't want to do.
- Try to be cognizant of power dynamics; one person shouldn't always be giving in or feeling like they're the only one who ever compromises.

- Only call each other by names that they like to be called; this means no name-calling and no using nicknames that the other person doesn't like.

- Are safe with one another and are never violent (no hitting, slapping, or punching). As your teen or young adult begins to hang out with crushes, date, or get into relationships, talk with them about dating abuse—that they deserve to be treated with kindness, and that they should come to you with any concerns about aggression or violence.

Many of these conversations come up naturally. Your child may come home from school feeling sad one day, sharing that someone who they thought was their friend ruthlessly made fun of them in front of others. Another day, they may be in high spirits because their friends remembered their birthday and decorated their locker in celebration. Listen to their feelings, be there with support and encouragement, and model what care and love look like. Encouraging your child to listen to their own feelings can also help them identify how they feel around friends and/or dating partners. Acknowledge when your child notices and describes their feelings ("I love hearing how happy you felt to go out with your friends today!") and model how you notice your own feelings ("I'm feeling sad because I learned today that one of my friends is really sick.").

Because all friendships and relationships have their ups and downs, try talking about healthy and unhealthy moments as compared with patterns. Even the healthiest relationships will have difficult moments; it's when these moments turn into patterns that it becomes problematic (or when the difficult moments are severe, such as being hit or sexually assaulted). You can also lead by example and show that, when we do mess up in a relationship, we give a sincere apology and try to do better. As an example: "I'm sorry I yelled at you; I was feeling scared when you weren't home by curfew and I lost my cool. I could have shared my concerns with you while still treating you with respect. Can we please start over? I'd love to hear more about your night."

"Catching Feelings"

Some people treat emotional intimacy and love as if they're diseases to avoid at all costs—even using the term "catching feelings" to describe the experience of developing an emotional attachment to another person. Indeed, every semester that I teach, young men write in their papers that they "feel different from other guys" because they want to find someone to fall in love with, often describing how lonely it feels for them to hook up with people they don't know well. They're surprised to hear that most people of all genders and sexual orientations (including most men) want love and connection. Girls just more often feel comfortable saying so, as they tend to be socialized to be nurturing and to desire love.

Given how much media coverage hookup culture gets, it's up to parents to counter it with facts: studies find that most teenagers (and adults too) prefer dating to casual hookups. Most people want to like someone who likes them back and even to fall in love—not just in the distant future, but sooner rather than later. And feeling emotionally connected to one's partner helps sex feel more fun, pleasurable, and arousing. Feelings matter. It's not love and emotional intimacy that are weird; what's weird is that love and emotional intimacy are treated as if they belong only to girls and women, rather than to all of humanity.

Power and Control

Just as it helps to disentangle sex from consent, it's also important to disentangle sex from issues of power and control. As you talk with your child about healthy relationships, consider how power is used within your own family. Families are children's earliest experiences of what it means to be in a relationship with other human beings. Here are some unhealthy ways that power and control are sometimes communicated in families:

- "I'm your parent and I know what's best for you."
- "I pay the bills, so I make the rules."
- "Finish every last bite or you can't have dessert."

These are one-sided uses of power. They don't involve communication or negotiation, nor do they suggest that the parent trusts their child or honors how they feel in their own bodies. And they can convey that the person who is the biggest or oldest, who acts aggressive, or who has the most money sets the rules.

Instead, try to convey the value of listening to one another, sharing power, and respecting people's expertise about themselves:

- "You know yourself better than anyone; I trust you to make this choice."
- "I need to keep you safe from _____. Can you tell me some ways to help you stay safe that work for you?"
- "I'm feeling worried about you doing that, but I also want to support you. Can you help me understand more about your idea?"
- "I love that you listened to your gut and left the party when you felt uncomfortable."
- "That's a difficult decision. How will you figure it out?"
- "You don't seem as happy lately. Can you help me understand more about what's going on and how you're feeling these days?"

Young people are trying to figure out so many parts of their lives—friendships, family relationships, romantic crushes or dating, gender and/or sexual identity, school, jobs, and their futures. As parents, we want to protect our children, but we also need to find places where we can let go of some control, especially when a decision is not likely to have major consequences. Giving kids space to make low-stakes decisions gives them opportunities to succeed and feel capable or, alternatively, to make and learn from their mistakes with only minor repercussions. When the stakes are higher, we may need to step in to share more of the decision-making or set a firm boundary, such as negotiating rules about technology use.

Breakups and Rejection

Nearly everyone will, at some point, get their heart broken or break someone else's heart. And nearly everyone who asks others out or expresses their interest in or feelings of love for another person will, at some point, be turned down. It hurts to be rejected (especially repeatedly or in a public way), and young people often wonder if anyone will ever fall in love with them. It's important to help your child develop skills to weather difficult experiences.

Young people need to know that:

- **Rejection, unrequited liking/love, and breakups happen to everyone.** Studies show that more than 90 percent of people have had their heart broken by the time they're in college, and the numbers only climb from there. On the bright side, this means these are common experiences, and so young people often have more support available to them than they may realize. Their parents, siblings, and friends can likely all relate.
- **It's okay to cry.** Expressing feelings is healthy; bottling up emotions is not. Boys and young men, especially, need to be supported in expressing their feelings. None of this "boys don't cry" or "man up" stuff. Everyone has feelings; sharing those feelings and asking for help getting through a difficult time are signs of strength, not weakness.
- **People deserve to be set free with kindness and compassion.** Even though rejection is hard, hearing the news directly is kinder than hearing through a friend or being ignored. When your child wants to break up with someone, delivering the news over the phone or in person is more compassionate than via texting or social media. Yes, it can be painful and anxiety producing to tell someone you're not into them. However, it's on the level of healthy stress—difficult

but not a tragedy—and getting practice managing healthy stress makes people stronger, more capable, and more confident over time. Encourage your child to rehearse with a parent, sibling, or close friend, if it would be helpful.

- **Some connections last hours and others last years, but each one is valuable.** After the initial pain has subsided, and if they're feeling ready, try to talk with your child about what they learned about themselves or about dating or love or affection from their time with the other person.

- **Rejection is not personal, even though it can feel that way.** Let your child know that when someone says no to a date or that they need to end a relationship, their choice is about themselves and not your child. Even though it may not feel like it at the time, rejection is a gift because the person is letting your child know not to waste their precious time, affection, or attention on them any longer.

- **There's no use trying to convince someone to stay.** Some people beg, plead, and promise to change just to get the other person to stay. Yet, it's better to gracefully accept the breakup. One can say, "I don't want to break up, but I accept your decision" or "Thanks for letting me know; I'm sad but I'll be okay." Sometimes breakups come as a surprise, and people react in ways they later regret (yelling, screaming, saying extreme things like "I can't live without you"). If that happens, rehearse a response with your child and encourage them to text their ex with something like, "I'm sorry I reacted the way I did. Although I'm sad, I accept the breakup and I wish you well" (or whatever feels true, more mature than their initial response, and will help them move on).

- **Some people react badly to being broken up with or rejected.** Ask your child to let you or another trusted adult know if they are concerned that the person they're cutting ties with may become abusive or violent, or if the other person is threatening self-harm or to hurt them.

If your child is prone to depression or anxiety, offer extra emotional support in the weeks and months following a breakup, which can feel like a profound loss. Your child may benefit from stepping away from social media, where they may be obsessively looking for signs of their ex moving on. Helping them to find new ways to fill their time might be healing: a long weekend away with family, taking up a new hobby, visiting relatives, or reconnecting with friends who got sidelined during the relationship. If your child is prone to aggression or violence, then, in addition to offering emotional support, you may need to seek professional support for them or monitor them more closely (including spot checks on their online behavior) to ensure they're not stalking or harassing their ex or planning to harm anyone.

Finally, offer hugs and undivided attention. Listen without judging. (And try to avoid speaking poorly of your child's ex, as they may end up back together.) Young love may differ from adult love, but it is still love. And tween and teen crushes have a special quality that is all their own, a newness that nothing else that comes later can quite replicate. Honor your child's crushes and relationships for what they are. Their feelings are real; respect and try not to trivialize their loss.

SEXUAL EXPLORATION

It's common for kids to explore their own bodies and to wonder about sexual behavior, whether in the context of making babies, expressing love, or experiencing pleasure. Here are some common topics that children either ask about or that you may want to address at some point.

Masturbation

There's a saying that sexuality is with us "from womb to tomb." Even infants and toddlers touch their own genitals, likely out of curiosity and/or pleasure.[15] Vulvas and penises are, after all, sensitive body parts; touching them helps us map out our bodies and understand what's what. Indeed, there's nothing wrong or unhealthy about self-exploration at any age, from infancy through old age. Masturbation won't make people go blind or grow hair on their palms. Still, it's wise to encourage children to limit this behavior to a private setting so that they don't masturbate in the family room or at school. If you find your child masturbating in common areas of your home, say, "That's fine to do, and I know it can feel good, but it's for a private area like your bedroom or the bathroom." If your child tends to need more direct instructions, clarify that it's "something you do when you are alone in your bedroom or alone in the bathroom at home." This may reduce the likelihood of socially awkward situations, such as masturbating in the school bathroom.

If your family has set boundaries in support of privacy, knock before entering your child's room. If you forget to knock and then walk in on them masturbating, apologize for entering their room without knocking and walk out. If your older teen or young adult child masturbates in a way that infringes on others' space—say, they're alone in their room but being loud (such as by audibly using a vibrator or watching sexually explicit media)— acknowledge their right to privacy alongside the rest of the family's right not to hear the details.

If your child has a disability and needs a personal care attendant for bathroom needs, the bathroom may not feel like a private option for them; in these cases, say, "That's fine to do, but wait until you are somewhere safe and private, such as your bedroom when you're the only one there." Also, let them know that if they need privacy from caregivers, they can ask for time alone.

As your child grows older, share that not only is masturbation common (in fact, it is the most common form of sex) and a healthy way of experiencing pleasure, but that it's also common whether people are single or in relationships. Some people masturbate more often when they have an active partnered sex life, and others masturbate less often under those circumstances. Also, people masturbate for many reasons—for pleasure as well as to learn about their body, to relieve stress, to fall asleep, or because they're bored. Everyone is different. Some transgender teens don't want to see or touch their chest or genitals whereas others may feel that exploring their changing body (such as from hormone treatment) helps them feel affirmed in their gender expression and happier in their own skin. Give your child the space to figure out what works for them.

While most people use their hand(s) to masturbate, some rub against blankets, pillows, or other objects, or (as older adolescents or young adults) use vibrators or other sex toys. Some of my college students have shared that, while growing up, they "borrowed" their parent's vibrator, without their knowledge. If you think your teen may be borrowing your vibrator, it's time to revisit conversations about boundaries and perhaps even get them their own.

If you describe masturbation as healthy but private, then you've set a foundation for later conversations about what to say or do if a friend, partner, or someone they chat with online one day asks them to take and send pictures or video of themselves masturbating. Girls, especially, are often pressured to send such pictures, often to teenage boys or adult men. Be clear that, in most places, it is illegal to take, share, or possess nude pictures of minors (see Chapter 5). Emphasize, too, that even if they fully trust their partner not to show the image to other people, many times it is that person's friends who find and pass along the images.

Finally, although most people masturbate, not everyone does. Some people mistakenly believe that all boys masturbate, and that's not true. Some people have no desire to masturbate. Others have tried masturbating and have just not been into it. Also, some people avoid masturbation for religious or cultural reasons, even if the desire is there. No one should feel pressured to have sex they're not into, and that includes masturbation.

Vibrators and Sex Toys

Don't be surprised if your teenager asks you to buy them a vibrator. Because vibrators make it easier to experience orgasm (and are used by more than half of adult women), they are often promoted in magazine articles and social media videos. Vibrators are also no longer relegated to adult stores; they are now widely available in stores as personal care items, and some teenage girls even give each other vibrators as gifts. Increasingly, parents describe being asked for a vibrator by their ten- to twelve-year-old daughters. If this happens to you, consider asking your child what they have heard about vibrators or where they've come across them. Often, it reflects a child having come across pornography. Learning this information helps some parents to step back and to steer the conversation away from "should I buy my kid a vibrator?" toward age-appropriate conversations about bodies, sexual exploration, pleasure, orgasm, and the fact that pornography is for adults (not kids). Parents can also validate their child's interest in self-pleasure, affirm that masturbation is normal and healthy, but encourage them to explore their body on their own for a while, delaying vibrator exploration until they're older.

However, just as every person is different, reasons for wanting to use a sex toy vary too. For some disabled teens and young adults, those who have undergone pelvic radiation, and/or young people whose sensory issues require more intense stimulation to experience genital arousal or orgasm, a vibrator or other sex toy may help them explore their bodily response in ways that their own hand doesn't. Also, people who find it difficult to ejaculate often require intense stimulation to experience orgasm. And for some, it's just about pleasure or variety.

Sexual Pleasure

Sexual pleasure and enjoyment are rarely addressed in high school sexuality education, which often focuses on pregnancy and STI risks as well as sexual assault prevention. This paints an incomplete picture of sex and makes some young people distrust adults, wondering why adults don't often acknowledge the upsides to sex. Try to give your child a holistic and balanced perspective on sexuality that addresses its risks as well as its rewards. Even for younger kids, you can share that people aren't usually having sex to make a baby but because it feels good or is a way that grown-ups sometimes express their romantic feelings or love for one another. As kids grow older, share that sex generally feels better when people know each other well, are in a relationship, care about one another, and/or are excited to have sex together.

It's important for young people to hear that sexual enjoyment matters. This is especially true for girls and young women and anyone who may be marginalized due to their gender, (dis)abilities, body size, or anything that makes them feel different. Be clear that your teen or young adult's sexual pleasure, joy, and dignity matter—whether in hookups or relationships. Also, make sure that your teen or young adult understands the ethics of treating sexual partners with kindness and respect, and that if they don't care about their partner's pleasure, they shouldn't be with them.

Orgasm

As your child moves into adolescence, there are many opportunities to relay information about orgasm thanks to magazine covers that promise mind-blowing orgasms and movies that joke about faking them. Share that:

- Learning to experience orgasm takes time, especially for cisgender women, who tend to experience their first orgasm in their teens, twenties, or beyond. In contrast, cisgender boys tend to experience their first orgasm around puberty, assuming their families have not been overly prohibitive about them masturbating. (Less is known about how orgasm unfolds for gender-diverse kids.) That said, some people start having orgasms at earlier ages and some at later ages.

- It's not unusual for orgasms to take an hour or so to experience in those early stages of learning, especially for people with vulvas. Orgasms often become easier and quicker with practice.

- Although orgasms can feel different from person to person, they usually feel like a discreet event—a pleasurable buildup that may last for a while followed by a mild or intense burst. Some people notice muscular contractions around their genitals or "see stars" (sparkly dots that are visual effects from brain-related processes involved in orgasm) when they experience orgasm; others do not.

- Teenagers and young adults with penises may ejaculate very quickly when they're making out or having sex with a partner. This is sometimes called *premature ejaculation* or *rapid ejaculation*. People usually learn to delay ejaculation with time and experience. Masturbation exercises like the stop-start technique can also help people learn to delay ejaculation; this involves stimulating the penis to a highly aroused state and then stopping stimulation, letting arousal decrease, then starting again.

- Orgasms are easier for people when they feel safe, comfortable, relaxed, and (for partnered sex) when they're with a relationship partner who cares about their pleasure. Orgasms are much less common with hookup partners.[16]

- Most people first experience orgasm during masturbation, when one can take time to touch, explore, and fantasize. In contrast, partnered sex makes some people feel pressured to perform, which can make orgasm difficult.

- No one should feel like they have to pretend to have an orgasm just to prop up their partner's ego or get them to finish.

- Orgasms are usually fun, pleasurable, and feel good—but this isn't always the case. Painful ejaculation can be a side effect of certain medications, including some antidepressants. Also, feeling pressured by a partner to have an orgasm can make people feel like something is wrong with them for not having an orgasm, or not having one quickly.[17]

Finally, teens and young adults need to hear that orgasm can occur even when a person is being sexually assaulted. Some people who have been assaulted feel confused by their body's orgasmic response, so let's be clear: an orgasm does not make an assault any less real. The vagina can lubricate due to arousal but also in a way that scientists think is simply protective (the idea being that if sex is happening or looks like it could happen, even without consent, then it's better for the body to start lubricating to reduce the risk of vaginal tearing or injury).[18] Orgasms and ejaculation can occur from vulvar and prostate stimulation even when that stimulation is unwanted or nonconsensual.

Sexual Orientation

Diverse sexual orientations may come up in many families' lives, especially as most people have LGBTQ+ friends and/or family members or watch shows with LGBTQ+ characters. Also, about one in six teenagers identify as LGBTQ+ (although not all are out to their family) and, regardless of how they identify, more than 10 percent of teens have had a same-sex sexual experience.[19]

In some ways, young people today are growing up in a more accepting society. According to a 2022 Gallup poll, nearly three-quarters of US adults now support marriage equality (same-sex marriage rights).[20] And a 2022 American Library Association survey found that most public school parents agree that age-appropriate books that address LGBTQ+ issues should be available in libraries.[21] However, LGBTQ+ harassment, discrimination, and violence remain prevalent and LGBTQ+ rights issues are too often politicized. Accordingly, numerous studies have shown that family support and acceptance are critical for LGBTQ+ youth. Being a loving, supporting, and accepting parent can significantly reduce a child's risk of mental health problems, substance use, and suicidal ideation.

If your child comes out to you as LGBTQ+, thank them for telling you and say, "I love you and I always will." Do not dismiss your child's identity or try to change it. Ask your child what kind of support they need from you—whether with family, friends, their school, your family's place of worship, or healthcare providers. And do what you can to broadcast love and to help combat discrimination in your community. Showing up to support your child and their friends, with pride and love, can be a lifeline.

For more information about LGBTQ+ lives or terminology, check out some of the websites listed in the **Resources** section.

Partnered Sex

Asking how babies are made is among childrens' earliest questions that lead to conversations about partnered sex. At older ages, they may begin asking questions about oral sex—perhaps phrased as "Why do people lick vaginas?" or "What's a blow job?" Often these are phrases they've heard at school; they may sense that older kids know something they don't, and they want to be in on the joke or the conversation. Questions like these are most common after age ten, but they begin earlier for some and later for others.

However, the longer you wait to directly answer their questions (or broach the topic if they haven't asked yet), the more likely it is that a friend may fill them in, they'll search the internet for information, or they'll be vulnerable to being taking advantage of. Young people also get inaccurate information about sex from friends, dating partners, social media, and movies, and sharing fact-based information with your child may help protect them from harm. If you can, introduce these topics yourself so that they can learn in a safe, loving, and supportive family context. When it's appropriate for your child's age and developmental stage, share that there are many ways that people are sexual together. Some of this involves kissing (with an open or closed mouth) as well as more intimate sexual behaviors such as oral sex, vaginal sex, and anal sex.

If your tween or teen has stumbled upon pornography, then they likely already know about diverse kinds of sex but could benefit from context. Young people don't often know how to understand what they've seen. They may wonder: *Are penises really that big? What is that fluid shooting out of the vagina or penis? Why doesn't my body look like that?* And since pornography often highlights aggressive sex, they may walk away with the idea that oral sex is aggressive, that intercourse is something one primarily does with strangers, or that most people like being called names like "slut" or "whore." (There's much to be said on this topic, which is why Chapter 6 is dedicated to addressing pornography.)

Focus on what you want your child to know about the many ways that people express themselves sexually. For a lot of parents, these are among the messages they wish to share:

- **There are many ways that people have sex.** It's common to explore on one's own (through masturbation) as well as with a partner to find out what feels good, both physically and in terms of what helps them feel cared for, comfortable, or loved. Exploring with a partner is usually done when someone is an older teenager or young adult (some families may say this occurs only after marriage). Explain what oral sex, vaginal sex, and anal sex are (when it's age-appropriate for your child to hear) and that some kinds of sex vary based on their partner's gender or how their body works. Share that there is no single type of sex that everyone is into or participates in, and that people can say no to anything they don't want to try.

- **Sex shouldn't hurt.** Say, "If sex hurts, let me know and I will help you." And, that sex that starts slow, is gentle, and is with someone a person knows well and with whom they can be vulnerable (without fear of being treated poorly) often makes for better sex. Taking time to build arousal before vaginal intercourse begins often makes it feel more comfortable; also, lubricant helps both vaginal and anal intercourse.

- **Most sex is not "mind blowing"**—no matter what magazines say or pornography suggests. It should ideally be fun, connecting, and help people feel good (at least most of the time). However, even happy, sexually satisfied couples sometimes have sex that is just so-so. Open communication, kindness, and listening to one another's sexual desires make for better sex.

- **If they're going to have penile-vaginal intercourse, even for a few seconds, they should use birth control or they could become pregnant.** Even the first time they have sex. And even if a person hasn't yet had their first menstrual period, as ovulation starts before the first period.
- **STIs can be passed through oral sex, vaginal sex, and anal sex, as well as through sharing of sex toys.** Some STIs can be passed even if a condom is used. (See Chapter 3.)

As many teenagers and young adults explore their gender and sexual orientation, talk with your child about sex in ways that help them feel seen, loved, and included—no matter how they end up identifying. Try not to make assumptions about their sexual orientation and what that may mean about their sexual behavior. Although some asexual people never have partnered sex, some do. And just as not all heterosexual people are into penile-vaginal intercourse, not all gay men are into anal sex. Sexual expression is diverse and fascinating; people vary.

Healthy Sexuality

As parents, we teach kids about bodies and sexuality because we want to help them develop a healthy expression of sexuality—one that brings them pleasure and fulfillment and does not harm other people. This involves thinking and talking about:

- **Consent,** which is the bare minimum expectation for sex to proceed.
- **STI and pregnancy prevention,** which can help people understand what kinds of risks they are taking when deciding to have sex, as well as how they can protect themselves and their partner(s).
- **Power and how it is used in their flirtations and sexual encounters;** this includes being aware of whether they may be taking advantage of others (or being taken advantage of).

- **Honesty.** This includes being honest about one's STI/HIV status (see Chapter 3), whether one is single or in a relationship, and one's hopes or intentions. Are both people interested in dating or a potential relationship? Or is this a casual hookup?
- **Mutual pleasure.** This means noticing (and sharing with their partner) what they like (or don't like) and what they want to try or avoid, checking in with one another ("How does that feel?"), and spending time together afterward to share feelings and address any discomfort.

You may have other ideas to share with your child. Some parents emphasize the value of being in a loving, committed relationship or of having sex only in a committed context, such as marriage. Some parents encourage their child to think about authenticity: To what extent do they feel like they can be themselves when it comes to their sexuality? Some talk with their teens about sexual integrity, which can involve applying values such as kindness, compassion, or generosity in one's relationships and sexuality. Ultimately, as your child moves into adulthood, they will decide what feels like healthy sexuality for them; however, bringing up these ideas earlier can act as a guidepost.

Collective Wisdom

So much of the knowledge and skills that support teens and young adults in creating safer, consensual, and pleasurable intimate experiences starts with what they learn as they are growing up.

1. **Teach kids about their bodies.** This includes how they work, and that they are incredible and deserve to be cared for, protected, and treated with respect.
2. **Talk about consent, boundaries, and power apart from sex.** If we want our teens and college-aged kids to understand consent and take it seriously, we need to build those muscles early on.

3. **Emphasize that people are the rulers of their own bodies—full stop.** They decide who touches them, they decide what is pleasurable, and they can say "no" or "stop" or "not like that" without having to give a reason. A "no" should always be respected.

4. **Help them identify what healthy friendships and relationships look and feel like.** They should feel safe, good inside, and that they can be themselves.

5. **Embrace the fact that nearly everyone wants emotional connection and intimacy.** Normalize the idea that feelings are for everyone, not just one gender.

3

Sexual and Reproductive Health

S exual and reproductive health is an important part of life, and as children grow up, they take on increasing levels of responsibility for it: scheduling gynecological exams, talking with healthcare providers about birth control or painful sex, finding affordable STI testing, or buying their own period products or condoms. Encourage your child to take on some of these tasks (if relevant to them) before they leave home for college, a gap year, or a job. After all, eventually they will need to make their own medical appointments and advocate for their health.

Unintended pregnancies have decreased in recent years, largely due to greater access to highly effective contraceptive methods such as implants and intrauterine devices (IUDs), but they remain prevalent. In many countries, more than 40 percent of pregnancies are unintended each year. For those younger than twenty years old, most pregnancies are unintended—as many as 70 to 80 percent in some places. In about half of unintended pregnancies, a person became pregnant not because they or their partner forgot to use birth control, but because the contraceptive didn't work. No method of birth control is perfect, though some are more effective than others.

On the other hand, STI rates keep rising, as too few people use condoms or seek STI testing and treatment. Each year, about one-quarter of teens will acquire an STI. Unfortunately, teens often make it through high school with little to no sexual health education that addresses condoms and how to use them, birth control, STI prevention and testing, sexual pleasure, painful sex, reproductive health, or LGBTQ+ health. Young people in special education often get even less in terms of sexuality information.

Well-meaning parents often believe (or hope?) that they have more time than they do before their child becomes sexually active. And many teachers who overhear school gossip about who's hooking up with whom are either not trained to deliver sex education or not permitted to answer students' sex questions. This chapter provides an overview of sexual and reproductive health information that is vital to young people's health but often missing from school-based sex education, leaving it to parents to fill in the gaps. It's wise to start talking with your child about birth control, pregnancy, and STIs sooner rather than later. All too often, by the time a teenager learns basic safer sex information, they are already unexpectedly pregnant or have an STI. Even if you dread having a safer sex talk with your child, it's not as bad as you might think. The information that follows is part crash course and part cheering squad. I believe in you!

A Note About Language

In some places in this chapter—especially when writing about STIs—I use the terms "male" and "female." This reflects the fact that some STIs, such as chlamydia, can behave differently in bodies of people born with a penis versus those born with a vagina. Although older kids and teens who receive gender-affirming care may transition socially (change their name, pronouns, or how they present) or use hormonal treatments, gender-affirming surgeries involving the genitals are extremely rare for minors. All that said, I understand that *male* and *female* terms don't fit everyone (nor do terms like *vulva* and *penis*, as noted in Chapter 2), so please substitute with language that best supports your child.

VULVAR AND TESTICULAR SELF-EXAMS

Caring for one's sexual health includes becoming familiar with one's own genitals and one's own personal "normal." You may have already told your child, "You know your body best; please tell me if anything ever hurts or feels unusual." After all, there is no way to know if another person's body hurts or itches unless they tell us. Because the genitals are private and rarely seen by others, it's extra important for people to look at their own genitals from time to time to check for changes. Most lumps, bumps, freckles, and moles will be benign and nothing to worry about, yet still it's wise to bring any new developments to a healthcare provider's attention, just to be sure. Changes in genital skin color should also be mentioned to a doctor or nurse, as they may be signs of a skin condition that could be helped with medication or changes to bathing or other hygiene habits.

Testicular self-exams—which involve rolling one's testicles between the thumb and forefinger to check for lumps—are especially important between ages fifteen and forty, given the increased risk for testicular cancer at these ages. As you're teaching your child about caring for their body, make sure to address monthly vulvar or testicular self-examination. Some people don't want to look at their genitals, especially if they feel self-conscious about their penis size, worried that their labia (vaginal lips) are too large or asymmetrical, or dysphoric about their genitals. As a parent, you can explain the value of genital self-examination (especially for early detection of cancers) and share diagrams or print out information from trustworthy websites. However, it's ultimately up to your child as to whether they will incorporate self-exams into their self-care.

TIME ALONE WITH PEDIATRICIANS

If your child is between ten and eighteen, their pediatrician may ask you to step into the hallway for a few minutes while they have one-on-one time with your child. This is common practice and gives kids a chance to ask and answer questions about their health and body. When parents are in the room, the parent may often answer questions on behalf of their child and may not realize that their child can and should answer many healthcare questions for themselves. Having time alone gives kids space to realize, perhaps even with pride, that they can capably manage their healthcare visits. One-on-one time also offers kids opportunities to discuss concerns that they might not feel ready to bring up around a parent. While some questions may be about sexuality or STI testing, often they're about acne, their height, body odor, mental health, learning disabilities, or substance use.

Before green-lighting your child's time alone with their provider, ask your child how they feel about their doctor or nurse. As with any healthy relationship, your child should feel safe, respected, and good inside when they're around their provider. LGBTQ+ youth, especially, may be looking for signs that they will feel safe and respected. To find an LGBTQ+ affirming and knowledgeable provider in your area, search OutCareHealth.org or ask for recommendations in local LGBTQ+ family social media groups. After your child has had time alone with their pediatrician, ask how it went and how they felt about it, but try not to pry for specifics. Although laws vary, patient-provider health conversations are usually treated as confidential, except in certain cases (such as if a child has a life-threatening condition). It can be difficult to let go, but it is all part of your child becoming more independent.

There are rare exceptions when one-on-one time may not feel like the right fit; if your child has a history of sexual trauma or abuse, they may understandably hesitate to be alone in an exam room with a provider. If so, talk in advance both with your child and with their pediatrician to see if there's a way to make time alone more comfortable. You might ask for a nurse to be in the room, too, or you could stay nearby in the hallway. Or your child can skip time alone until they're more comfortable.

Meeting alone with one's provider is also key, because at some point (often around age eighteen) they will transition into adult care and need to take charge of their own healthcare, especially if they are moving away for college or a job. If your child feels attached to their pediatrician, let them know well in advance that they'll need to transition to a new provider. And if you have questions about one-on-one time, ask your child's healthcare provider at their next visit.

SHAME-FREE APPROACHES TO STIS

Just as you don't need to know everything about sex to be askable, you don't need to be a walking STI encyclopedia to be helpful to your child. It's a good idea to know some STI basics (which I'll share with you) as well as where to turn for detailed information (I've got you covered here too). Yet, STI facts are only one piece of the puzzle. One of the greatest STI-related gifts parents can give their kids (and yes, I contend there is such a thing) is the belief that having an STI does not make someone bad, dirty, or undesirable. More than half of people will have at least one STI by the time they're twenty-five, even if they don't realize it. Also, many people will have a partner with an STI—again, even if they don't realize it. Having an STI also does not mean a person is a "slut" (a term I keep hoping will go away). Having an STI simply means that a person is living in a world full of bacteria, viruses, and other organisms, some of which are passed through sexual behaviors. That's it. Just as having the flu or COVID is not a moral failure, neither is having an STI. Why is this an important message to share? Because when people attach shame and stigma to STIs, they may:

- Delay getting tested for STIs, including HIV.
- Hesitate to ask their partner if they've been tested for STIs.
- Feel bad about themselves if they have an STI, contributing to anxiety or depression.

- Avoid telling their partner they have an STI, for fear of being rejected or shamed.
- Say negative or judgmental things about STIs that keep their partner from sharing their own STI or HIV status.

STI-related shame can even keep people in abusive relationships. Some people have shared that they stayed with abusive partners because they had an incurable STI (such as herpes or HIV) and worried that no one else would want them or that having an STI made them "damaged goods." Sometimes those beliefs were shaped directly by their partner's abuse. Abusive comments regarding STIs ("Go ahead and leave me, do you think anyone else will want you now that you have herpes?") are meant to demean and isolate, and they may be more effective if someone already has underlying negative beliefs about people who have STIs.

Treating STIs as plain old infections rather than scarlet letters is good for us all. Try:

- **Saying that STIs are like other common infections, such as influenza (the flu).** STIs are nothing to be embarrassed about and should be part of family conversations about health. Just as you remind your child when it's time to get a flu shot, you can take the same casual tone in saying that it's time to get the HPV vaccine.
- **Standing up to STI jokes.** If your teen jokes about a peer having an STI, say, "STIs are very common. I don't know if this person has an STI or not but, if they do, they could use kindness. It takes courage for someone to tell friends or partners that they have an STI."
- **Learning about STIs.** Some people living with HIV describe having friends and family members refuse to hug them even though HIV is not transmitted via hugging, but rather through direct sexual contact such as unprotected intercourse. Gathering facts about STIs can help dispel myths, decrease fear, and increase acceptance.

- **Being risk aware but not risk focused.** Although sexual and gender minority youth are at greater risk for STIs, anyone can get infected. If you have more than one child and one identifies as LGBTQ+, don't just talk with your LGBTQ+ kid about safer sex or STIs (which is stigmatizing); make sure all your children of relevant age are part of those conversations.

When talking with your child about STIs, try not to freak them out. The goal is to support them—not terrify them. When I was a teenager, my classmates and I were shown pictures of vulvas and penises that were covered in warts or lesions. Decades later, my college students tell similar stories about their high school sex education. Yet, most people who have an STI have genitals that don't look anything like these worst-case images. Genital warts from HPV infection aren't always visible to the naked eye. Herpes is rarely visible except during outbreaks, which are infrequent, especially if a person is being treated. Extreme-case STI photos may create the false impression that a person can tell whether someone has an STI by inspecting their genitals or anus. Yet, most of the time a visual inspection won't reveal much except freckles or a birthmark. If someone wants to know if they or their partner has an STI, they should seek out STI testing.

STI vs. STD

In case you're wondering about the term *sexually transmitted infection* (STI), and whether it and *sexually transmitted disease* (STD) mean the same thing—in short, yes, both terms refer to having chlamydia, gonorrhea, HIV, syphilis, herpes, or a similar diagnosis. The term STI is often used in my field because (1) people who have STIs don't always develop symptoms, which means they don't reach a "diseased" state, and (2) some feel that the word *disease* is stigmatizing. That said, the term STI has yet to become commonplace, so use whichever term feels more comfortable.

STI BASICS

There are two main types of STIs—those caused by bacteria (including chlamydia, gonorrhea, syphilis, and *Mycoplasma genitalium*) and those caused by viruses (including HPV, herpes, and HIV)—though there are others we'll cover too. My students find it helpful to think about STIs in these bacterial and viral buckets because it helps them remember that some STIs (the bacterial ones) can often be cured and other STIs (the viral ones) may be treated but tend to stick around, even if they don't show symptoms.

The fact that some STIs can be cured is exciting news to many people, who often feel worn down by scare tactics from their school's sex education. Across generations, many people have summed up their family or high school sex education as, "If you have sex, you will get an STI and die." Those of us who grew up in the early days of the HIV epidemic recognize a grain of truth in this, because we remember all too well when large numbers of young, healthy people—mostly young gay and bisexual men—did get sick and die of HIV/AIDS-related medical conditions. It was an awful time, where the death toll was made worse by fear, homophobia, and stigma that stalled needed investment in prevention, treatment, and care. But this is not the 1980s or 1990s, and HIV can now be managed successfully. When people with HIV are connected to care and treatment, they often live a typical lifespan.

Hearing that some STIs can be cured is enough for some young people to feel like STIs are not all doom and gloom and that getting tested for STIs is a good idea. Even if someone learns they have chlamydia or syphilis, they can feel optimistic that antibiotics will cure the infection. It's also important for young people to understand that not all STIs can be cured and that some do persist in the body; that way, they can make thoughtful, informed choices about sex.

While I share key information below about common STIs to support conversations within your family, if you're interested in learning more, visit CDC.gov and search for their STD fact sheets. And if you really want to geek out on STIs, check out Dr. Ina Park's funny and smart book *Strange Bedfellows: Adventures in the Science, History, and Surprising Secrets of STDs*.

Bacterial STIs

Bacterial STIs include chlamydia, gonorrhea, syphilis, and *Mycoplasma genitalium* (MG). These can be passed through unprotected oral, vaginal, and anal sex (as well as through sharing sex toys), and they especially impact teenagers and young adults. STIs can also be transmitted to a baby during childbirth, which is why healthcare providers often test for STIs during pregnancy.

Chlamydia is the most common bacterial STI. People can pass chlamydia even if they don't ejaculate during sex, as it can be passed via pre-ejaculate (pre-cum). Chlamydia is often asymptomatic. When people do notice symptoms, these may include vaginal or penile discharge, a burning sensation while peeing, or rectal pain. (Even if a person has never had anal intercourse, they can still get rectal STIs, though exactly how this happens is not well understood.[22]) Untreated chlamydia can lead to pelvic inflammatory disease and infertility, making regular STI testing important. Fortunately, using a condom reduces the risk of transmission; also, chlamydia can be cured with antibiotics.

Next up is **gonorrhea**, which frequently shows no symptoms for females but often does for males, who may notice discharge from their penis or a burning sensation while peeing. For females, symptoms may include increased vaginal discharge, bleeding in between periods, or a burning sensation while peeing. However, some people mistake these symptoms for other causes, leading to delays in them seeking out STI testing. I remember one teenage girl who, although she had noticed increased vaginal wetness, assumed she was extra lubricated because she'd been feeling aroused lately. Having an STI hadn't even crossed her mind. For gonorrhea affecting the anus, symptoms include anal itching, discharge, soreness, bleeding, and painful bowel movements. Gonorrhea can be prevented through condom use and can often be cured with antibiotics. However, some gonorrhea strains are resistant to antibiotics and difficult to treat. This underscores how helpful using a condom can be, especially with a new partner or one whose STI status is unknown.

Syphilis is another bacterial STI that can be cured with antibiotics. Condoms can reduce the risk of transmission, but if a person has a syphilis lesion in an area not covered by the condom (such as the pubic mound, the triangular area where pubic hair grows), then the infection can still be passed. Syphilis is more common among men who have sex with men, but anyone can get it. Sores are a common early symptom. If syphilis is untreated, symptoms may include a rash, fever, sore throat, hair loss, headaches, and/ or fatigue. Although syphilis can be deadly if untreated, it's almost always treated in earlier stages, making it extremely rare for people to die of it today.

Mycoplasma genitalium **(MG)** is an STI that few have heard of even though it's been recognized by scientists for decades. MG is most often spread through vaginal and anal sex. Although it can affect people of any gender and sexual orientation, MG is more common among men who have sex with men. When it shows symptoms at all, they're similar to chlamydia symptoms. Because MG can be resistant to antibiotics (and its more effective treatments can cause serious side effects), many healthcare providers don't recommend routine screening or treatment for MG unless a person is symptomatic. If most doctors don't test for it outside of research studies, why bother mentioning it? If a person has genital symptoms (recurrent vaginal bleeding, discharge, or genital irritation, especially urethral irritation in males) but tests negative for the usual suspects like chlamydia and gonorrhea, it can be helpful to ask a healthcare provider if MG could be a possibility.

Viral STIs

Viral STIs can also be passed through oral, vaginal, and anal sex (as well as through sharing sex toys). The most common viral STI is **human**

papillomavirus (HPV). HPV doesn't usually show noticeable symptoms. While it cannot be cured, it can go dormant and does not usually cause major problems. Some HPV strains cause genital warts, which are painless and often too tiny to see with the naked eye. Some look like small pimples; others are larger and cauliflower shaped. Still, they often resolve on their own or can be treated. Other HPV strains cause cervical changes that may show up on a Pap test. Rarely, HPV can lead to cancer of the cervix, vulva, penis, anus, head, or neck. Fortunately, most of the time, HPV infection clears on its own, especially for those with healthy habits (getting good sleep, eating fruits and vegetables, not smoking).

As of this writing, the CDC recommends HPV vaccination for eleven- and twelve-year-olds of all genders; ask your child's pediatrician for more information. Young adults who didn't get the HPV vaccine as kids can still get vaccinated as teens or young adults (again, they should check with their provider). You may be thinking, *Why eleven or twelve? My child won't be having sex at that age!* While it's true that most young people don't have sex until much later, some will, and it's not easy to know who will and who won't. Also, there is the unfortunate reality that some children will be sexually assaulted. About 17 percent of high school girls and 5 percent of boys have been sexually assaulted, with LGBTQ+ youth more often impacted (22 percent of LGBTQ+ youth versus 9 percent of heterosexual youth have been sexually assaulted).[23]

Studies are clear that getting the HPV vaccine does not make kids jump into sex. But when young people do eventually become sexually active, they'll be better protected if they've been vaccinated. Condoms offer some protection from HPV, although it's more limited as HPV can live in skin in areas not covered by a condom. Still, condoms are an excellent choice for vaginal intercourse, to protect the cervix from potential HPV infection.

Another common STI is **herpes,** which is caused by HSV-1 (usually affects the mouth) or HSV-2 (usually affects the genitals). Herpes cannot be cured but can be treated, which may reduce the frequency and severity of outbreaks as well as reduce the likelihood of transmission to partners.

Thanks to changes in people's sexual behaviors as well as greater use of effective medications,[24] rates of genital herpes have been declining. Yet, it remains common, with about 12 percent of people having genital herpes (and around half of people having HSV-1, usually on the mouth). People can transmit herpes to one another even if they don't have an active outbreak at the time. Condoms offer some but not total protection from herpes.

The **human immunodeficiency virus (HIV)** is passed through semen, vaginal fluids, blood, and breast/chest milk. HIV is now largely considered a manageable infection; treatment is so effective that people can often reduce the amount of virus in their body to such a low point that their viral load may be described as undetectable. When a person's viral load is this low, the CDC indicates that there is likely no risk of transmitting HIV through oral, vaginal, or anal sex.[25] People with HIV often live a typical lifespan, though keeping the virus in check does involve taking medications, some of which may cause unpleasant side effects. Condoms are highly effective at protecting against HIV transmission as is PrEP (which stands for pre-exposure prophylaxis), pills or shots that people can take to prevent getting HIV if exposed. When used as prescribed, PrEP is highly effective against HIV transmission. However, people who take PrEP are wise to continue using condoms with new partners or those whose STI status is unclear, as people can still transmit other STIs.

The STI Misfits

Not all infections fit neatly into the bacterial and viral STI buckets. **Trichomoniasis** (called "trich") is caused by a parasite; symptoms in a female include vaginal irritation and/or a strong, fishy vaginal odor. Males usually have no symptoms; when they do, those may include a burning sensation while peeing or urethral irritation. Condoms reduce the risk of trich transmission. **Pubic lice** (called "crabs") are caused by a parasitic insect that has a penchant for pubic hair. When Brazilian waxing and other pubic hair removal trends became popular in the 2000s, pubic lice largely vanished, making occurrences rare today.[26] Pubic lice can be spread through sexual contact or by towels and bedding used by an infected person; when people have pubic lice, both their pubic hair and their bedding require treatment.

Other infections can sometimes be transmitted through sexual contact, too. Although the **Zika virus** is most often transmitted through mosquito bites and may be passed from a pregnant person to their fetus, there have been more than thirty documented cases of Zika being sexually transmitted (most often from men to women).[27] Then there's **mpox** (previously known as monkeypox), which, in July 2022 was declared a "public health emergency of international concern" by the World Health Organization. Mpox may be passed through close personal contact—especially skin-to-skin contact—making sex one route of transmission. Although mpox spread rapidly among men who have sex with men and was more common among those with multiple sex partners, it was not limited to either men or to LGBTQ+ individuals. Viruses don't care who you are; they care what you do. Mpox is a virus that thrives on close, prolonged skin contact. Vaccines can help to prevent mpox, as can limiting the number of one's sexual partners.

There are dozens more infections that may be sexually transmitted but are less common, have decreased given the availability of vaccines (like hepatitis A and B), or simply receive less attention (like hepatitis C, chancroid, scabies). That doesn't mean they aren't important. Encourage your child to take care of their body and to seek out medical care for any genital or anal itching, discharge, irritation, lesions, urethral irritation, or pain that does not go away.

NAVIGATING STIS WITH PARTNERS

Amsale and Bobby were two young men who were thinking about becoming sexually intimate when Bobby shared that he was HIV positive. To his credit, Bobby was forthcoming with Amsale about his HIV status, including sharing that his HIV had been effectively treated to the point where he had undetectable levels of virus and was thus unlikely to transmit HIV to others through sex. While that would be reassuring for some people, Amsale didn't feel comfortable having sex with Bobby due to his HIV status and turned Bobby down as a romantic partner. They agreed to try to remain friends and classmates, but shortly thereafter, Bobby filed a report on campus claiming that Amsale discriminated against him in violation of Title IX and other school discrimination policies not only by declining to have sex with him due to his HIV status, but also by sharing with friends that Bobby had HIV. Amsale sought Kristina and Susan's representation to find a way forward.

Bobby found it difficult to understand that Amsale had a right to consider infection status when deciding whether to engage in a sexual relationship with someone. He felt that, because his HIV viral load was so low, his HIV status should not have been a consideration for Amsale. At the same time, Bobby felt hurt that Amsale shared his HIV status with other people without his permission, after Amsale's friends had criticized his decision to reject Bobby.

Amsale recognized that going through a typical Title IX process would be exhausting, emotional, and expensive (as each had retained legal counsel). Neither wanted to share their personal details in a formal hearing, where each side would be subjected to lawyers testing their credibility through cross-examination, or with a formal university panel, which would ultimately decide whether there was a policy violation and potentially levy sanctions such as suspension or expulsion. Amsale and Bobby agreed to resolve the complaint through an informal resolution process, essentially a mediation, that resulted in an agreement that contained terms and conditions. Both students agreed to participate in sex education classes, refrain from talking about each other, and maintain a no-contact order.

When talking with your child, share that (1) it's important to be honest about one's STI/HIV status even if that means risking rejection; (2) it's okay to take a person's infection status into account when choosing whether to have sex with them; and (3) one should not disclose other people's health or medical information without their permission. Instead of sharing Bobby's HIV status with others, Amsale could have said, "We just weren't the right fit for one another," and left it at that.

Medical Conditions, Disabilities, and Sexuality

Millions of young people are affected by medical conditions and disabilities. Some conditions (or their treatment) affect sexuality. As examples: Diabetes can lead to less reliable erections. Both depression and some of the antidepressants used to treat it can cause low desire or difficulty reaching orgasm. Spinal cord injury can affect genital sensation, arousal, and time to orgasm (using a vibrator can help). Genital lichen sclerosus (a benign skin disorder often marked by white patches of skin and itching) can cause vulvar itching, difficulty retracting foreskin, or painful intercourse. Pelvic radiation can narrow the vagina, which may require parents to help young children use vaginal dilators to keep the vagina open and flexible. And while people who have a stoma (an opening in the abdominal area that allows urinary or fecal waste to leave the body) can have enjoyable sexual lives, lubricant may ease vaginal penetration as might exploring different sexual positions. Take note: Some people get curious and want to try to penetrate their partner's stoma, which can cause damage and spread STIs. Penetrating a stoma is not recommended.

If your teen or young adult has a disability, or if they have (or had) a medical condition that may affect their sexual lives, support their need for information about how to manage masturbation and/or sexual intimacy in safe and pleasurable ways. A member of their care team (pediatrician, recreation therapist, physical therapist) may be able to offer suggestions; also, sexuality-specific information is often available through patient-centered organizations and support groups.

PREGNANCY 101

Although most teenagers want to have kids one day, the key phrase is "one day" (often far in the future). To help your child understand how to prevent pregnancy, one first needs to understand how pregnancy happens—something many people (even adults) haven't always been taught. To become pregnant:

- Both an egg and a sperm are needed.
- The sperm and egg need to meet (when this happens via sex, they meet in the fallopian tube).
- The sperm must fertilize the egg.
- The fertilized egg has to successfully implant into the lining of the uterus (called the *endometrium*).

If a fertilized egg implants elsewhere (such as a fallopian tube), it's called an *ectopic implantation* (or *ectopic pregnancy*). This is a medical emergency, as it can cause the fallopian tube to burst and lead to life-threatening blood loss; pregnancy cannot progress in these cases.

Fertilization, and thus pregnancy, can happen at any time of the month. Although eggs are only viable for less than a day after being released from an ovary, some people ovulate more than once a month. Also, sperm can live inside a vagina and uterus for several days. This means that even if semen enters the vagina several days before ovulation, the sperm may survive long enough to find an egg and fertilize it. Scientists have found that there are no truly "safe" days in a menstrual cycle, which is why birth control is vital for sexually active people who wish to prevent pregnancy.

Understanding how pregnancy begins makes it easier to understand how birth control methods work and how to choose an effective one. Most methods prevent pregnancy by preventing ovulation. Hormonal birth control (the pill, patch, shot, ring, implant, some IUDs, and emergency contraception) all work this way. After all, if there's no egg, then even if sperm are ejaculated into the vagina, they won't find an egg to fertilize, and pregnancy won't occur. Some hormonal methods also thicken the cervical mucus, thus preventing sperm from reaching an egg should one be released, and/or thin the uterine lining, making implantation difficult. Barrier methods such as condoms and diaphragms prevent pregnancy by blocking sperm from getting into the uterus. If sperm can't reach the egg, then pregnancy cannot occur.

Gynecologic Care

Having one's first gynecologic exam is an important step in caring for one's sexual health; it's often recommended that gyn exams begin between ages thirteen and fifteen.[28] At these younger ages, the focus is on talking, establishing a patient-provider relationship, and giving teens a chance to ask questions about menstrual periods and their health. Healthcare providers may do a general exam (listening to the heart and lungs) and examine the vulva. However, there is usually no reason for a pelvic exam unless there's a medical need, such as if a teen reports unexplained vaginal bleeding or pelvic pain. Pelvic exams are more commonly offered to older teens and young adults, and/or once someone has been sexually active with a partner or has been sexually assaulted. Let your teen know that they can have you or another family member present at their exam if they would like, although they may prefer privacy, which should be respected. You might also ask your teen if they would prefer to have a provider of a certain gender/sex, of their same race or ethnicity, or who is known to be LGBTQ+ affirming. Where possible, try to find a good match for your teen.

BIRTH CONTROL METHODS

Most people will use some type of contraceptive method during their lifetime. Among sexually active fifteen- to nineteen-year-olds, about 80 percent report using some kind of birth control—but only 59 percent report using a highly effective method. And particularly worrisome, only three-quarters of teenage girls reported that they and their partner used any kind of contraceptive the first time they had penile-vaginal intercourse. Of those who did use a contraceptive, condoms were the method most often used. Most teens say that the main reason they don't use birth control is because they are afraid their parents will find out.[29] Yet, most parents report that, if their teenager were sexually active, they would want to know so they could ensure their teen was using birth control.

Here's what you need to know to have impactful conversations with your child about birth control. First, there are two broad categories of contraception: permanent (tubal ligation, vasectomy) and reversible (which one can stop and still be able to become pregnant). Most young people want a pregnancy at some point in their lives, and so we'll focus on reversible contraception here, though if your young adult child wants to explore permanent contraception, they should talk with their healthcare provider.* Among the reversible options, presented in order from most to least effective:[30]

- **Abstinence** is 100 percent effective at pregnancy prevention when people truly abstain from penile-vaginal intercourse. However, some people rub their penis and vulva together without penetration (outercourse), or they try intercourse "for just a minute" and get carried away—with ejaculation happening much more quickly than young people often expect. In these cases, abstinence may fail. But when abstinence is done perfectly, it works well—at least for pregnancy prevention. As for STI prevention, abstinence can be effective if people are abstaining from oral sex, vaginal sex, and anal sex, but researchers often find that young people abstain from one or two of these, but not all three, which introduces STI risks.
- **IUDs** and **implants** are the most effective forms of birth control (>99 percent effective), providing years of protection (the exact number of years depends on which brand is used). A healthcare provider places the IUD in the uterus or places the implant under the skin of the upper arm.
- The **birth control shot** is about 94 percent effective and is administered by a healthcare provider once every three months. Many

---

* Many healthcare providers won't offer permanent sterilization (tubal ligation or vasectomy) to young adults in case they later change their mind and wish to become pregnant; they often recommend long-lasting, highly effective methods such as IUDs or implants instead. If a person still wants sterilization, they should discuss their options with a healthcare provider.

people find that their periods stop in the first year of use; some like this, some do not.

- The **birth control pill** is more than 90 percent effective and is popular (likely because it's been around for more than sixty years and is highly effective), but there's more room for error since it involves having to remember to take a daily pill.

- The **birth control patch** and **birth control ring** have effectiveness rates similar to the pill, as they, too, involve people needing to remember to do something, such as change the skin patch or the vaginal ring on time.

- **Condoms** are very effective for pregnancy prevention; they'd be more effective if more people used them correctly, including from start to finish during sex (taking a condom off midway through sex, as people do far too often, is not effective; neither is starting sex without a condom and adding one later). A huge upside of condoms is that they reduce STI/HIV risks. Condoms can also be used to "double up" protection with another method (like the pill, patch, IUD, or implant).

- **Withdrawal ("pulling out")** is moderately effective for pregnancy prevention. Some people have excellent ejaculatory control and consistently pull out prior to ejaculating. Others—especially young people who are new to sex—may be less reliable about pulling out on time. Plus, some people seem to "leak" sperm into their pre-ejaculatory fluids (pre-cum), and if those sperm find an egg, then fertilization and pregnancy may occur. Withdrawal is better than nothing, but it's better used to double up with another form of birth control than as stand-alone pregnancy prevention.

- **Fertility-awareness-based (FAB) methods** are less effective, with about one-quarter of women using these methods becoming pregnant within the first year of typical use. There are different approaches to FAB methods (tracking one's calendar, tracking temperature and/or vaginal discharge) and they can be complicated to do well. People who want to use FAB methods should talk with their healthcare provider for guidance. It's even more effective to pair FAB methods with another, more reliable method, such as condoms.

These aren't the only available reversible birth control methods (you may also be familiar with diaphragms, sponges, cervical caps, and spermicide), but they are the ones that teenagers and young adults use most often. The best method for your teen or young adult will be one that they can use consistently and correctly and that feels right with their body. Also, there are many reasons people use contraception that have nothing to do with sex, such as managing acne, endometriosis, menstrual migraines, or (for athletes) to time menstruation in relation to one's sport.

Finally, there's **emergency contraception (EC),** also called the *morning-after pill.* This name is a misnomer, as EC can be taken for up to five days after unprotected sex and can be taken any time of day or night. EC is highly effective and works primarily by delaying or preventing ovulation. However, EC should not be considered first-line birth control, as using a highly effective birth control method (pill, patch, shot, ring, IUD, implant) is more effective than tracking down and taking EC on an as-needed basis.

It's wise to start talking about birth control early as it takes time and repeated exposure to learn. Say, "When you are ready to become sexually active with a partner, I want you to know that you can come and talk with me. I will be happy to help you find a highly effective method of birth control and STI prevention." Share that you care about your child's health, you want them to have an enjoyable sex life (when it's time), and using highly effective methods to prevent pregnancy and STIs can help them reduce stress and enjoy intimacy.

I encourage you to talk about birth control with your child no matter what their gender or sexual orientation may be; young bisexual women and those questioning their sexual orientation are less likely to use birth control and, as a result, more often experience unintended pregnancy. Bisexual women also experience higher rates of sexual assault. If you're wondering how to approach your gay, lesbian, or asexual teen about birth control without making them feel like you're disrespecting their identity, here's one approach. As a college professor, I worry that some students will tune out the birth control lecture, if they expect to only have same-sex partners or don't plan to have vaginal intercourse for any number of reasons (like if they're not interested in sex or plan to abstain from sex until marriage). I ask my students of all sexual identities and sexual choices to pay close attention anyway. "Even if you don't think this information is relevant to you," I say, "having information about birth control may one day help a roommate, friend, or sibling." And indeed, more times than I count, that's what students tell me—that they have been able to jump in, correct others' misinformation, and steer friends and siblings toward healthcare providers and other trustworthy sources to learn about effective birth control methods or get EC when needed.

What Young People Want

Wondering what you can say or do to support your teen as they learn to care for their sexual health? Here are some things that, looking back on their adolescence or young adulthood, some people in research studies,[31] as well as my own students, say they wish their parents would have said or done:

- Said, "If you ever feel like you want to get on birth control, please come and talk with me. I'm here to help you."
- Described using birth control, or going on PrEP, as a responsible choice.
- Offered to make them an appointment for a gyn exam or to get birth control.
- Asked them if they feel respected and welcome at their healthcare provider's office and, if not, offered to help them find a better fit (especially important for LGBTQ+ youth).
- Asked their pediatrician's office to be more inclusive, such as by listing more options for gender and sexual identity on the intake form.

COMMON BIRTH CONTROL QUESTIONS

Most young people are interested in learning about condoms and other forms of birth control but have heard misinformation. Here are some common questions I hear from young people as well as some straightforward answers.

Q. Can you get pregnant during your period?

Yes. Ovulation can occur at any point in the month, and some people ovulate more than once in a given month. If a person does not want to become pregnant, they should use a highly effective form of birth control.

Q. Are two condoms better than one?

Nope! Using two condoms at once can cause friction and thus tearing. People should use one condom at a time.

Q. Is EC the same as an abortion pill?

No. EC prevents pregnancy by delaying or preventing ovulation (the release of the egg from the ovary). EC does not end pregnancy, but instead works to prevent pregnancy from happening in the first place.

Q. Is it safe to combine pill packs to skip my period?

Some people who use birth control pills choose to skip the last week of certain birth control pill packs (if using the kind without hormones in that week, which is sometimes called the "placebo week") and start a new pill pack right away. This can help them avoid menstrual migraines or skip their period while on vacation or for an athletic event. If your child wants to try this, they should ask their healthcare provider to make sure doing so will be safe and effective with their particular pill pack.

Q. Doesn't hormonal birth control cause side effects?

While some people experience side effects from hormonal birth control (pill, patch, ring, etc.), most either don't notice any side effects or else find that the side effects go away within a few months. If the side effects aren't horrible and your teen can stick it out to see if they go away, it could be worth it. If the side effects are uncomfortable or persist, checking in with one's healthcare provider is a good next step.

Q. Will birth control pills make me gain weight?

Studies have not found a link between birth control and weight gain, even though some people feel this happened to them. Because many people start birth control pills at young ages when their bodies are still developing, they may attribute weight gain to the pill rather than to maturing or changing their eating and exercise habits. The birth control shot, however, has been associated with slight weight gain during the first year, though some people may gain or lose weight differently.

Q. Can using birth control now hurt my fertility later on?

No. With the exception of surgical forms of contraception (sterilization), which are considered permanent, birth control methods are reversible. People can stop them at any time if they decide to try to become pregnant.

Anticipating Pregnancy Risk

Parents should talk with their child about pregnancy risk before they leave home to live on their own or head off to college, especially in places where abortion is illegal or severely restricted. These conversations should involve making sure that they: (1) understand the existing and proposed abortion laws, both civil and criminal, where they're moving to; (2) plan to bring EC and pregnancy tests with them; (3) understand highly effective forms of birth control (think: IUD and implant); and (4) know that, if there is any concern about pregnancy—even if remote—they should test early. If they wait too long, they may have too little time to seek abortion care, if wanted. Even those who don't expect to have penile-vaginal intercourse (or who only expect to have same-sex partners) should think through these issues given the possibility of sexual assault and, also, that people do sometimes get drunk or carried away and make different choices than they might when sober.

ERECTIONS

Many of my college students ask questions about erection problems, which some men and other people who have a penis are often surprised to experience at such a young age. I reassure them that erection difficulties are common, and erection difficulties are not the same as erectile dysfunction, which is rare among young, healthy men. Erection difficulties occur for various reasons, including feeling nervous, worrying about lasting long enough, drinking alcohol, recreational drug use, side effects from prescription medications (especially some used to treat depression or anxiety), or simply not feeling emotionally connected to or turned on by one's partner. And while condoms are great choices for reducing pregnancy and STI risk, some people find it difficult to maintain their erection while wearing a condom.

Just hearing that erection problems are common, normal, and not the same as erectile dysfunction is enough to relieve the pressure many people put on themselves. Here are some other suggestions to pass along (sticky note this page for your teen to find):

- **Choose partners you find emotionally and/or physically attractive.** This may sound obvious, but the pressure on young people (especially men) to have sex with whoever offers it to them is real. This is not a recipe for pleasurable sex or reliable erections. Men are sometimes embarrassed to admit that their erections are stronger and more reliable with relationship partners, but research studies back up that this is often the case. Try to normalize the fact that sex is indeed better for most people when their partner is someone they truly like and are into.

- **Involve your partner in condom use.** Want to be safe and still keep an erection? People can ask their partner to put the condom on their penis, which frees them to focus their attention on their partner as well as their own sexual arousal rather than fidgeting with a condom, which can be distracting. After the condom is on, they or their partner can place water-based lubricant on the outside of the condom. Because it feels good to have one's penis stroked, this can make their erection stronger. Bonus: lubricant helps make sex more comfortable and pleasurable for both partners.

- **Broaden your sex menu.** Sometimes penises just don't get or stay hard. That's okay. Fortunately, there are many kinds of pleasurable sex including oral sex, hand-genital stimulation, sex toy use, fingering, and making out. Moving on to sexual activities that don't require an erection can decrease pressure and increase pleasure.
- **Practice self-acceptance.** Bodies don't always work the way we want them to. People cannot become erect on demand (or lubricate on demand, for that matter). Erection problems don't make anyone less masculine, less sexy, or less of a sexual partner.
- **Reduce alcohol intake.** Erections tend to be stronger and more reliable when people are sober.

Finally, some people have heard rumors that watching pornography and/or masturbating can cause erectile dysfunction. Evidence for these ideas is lacking; however, some people prefer to set pornography and/or masturbation aside for a while and see how it feels. That's a personal choice. Just make sure your teen or young adult knows that masturbation is a healthy and common sexual behavior and nothing about which they should feel ashamed.

What Do I Say?

Talking About Sexual Health

Q. When should I talk with my kid about birth control and STIs?

It's never too early to introduce the idea of birth control. For many families, this comes up when children ask, "Are you going to have another baby?" Some parents answer this question by saying, "No, our family is complete; your father had a vasectomy," and then explaining what that means in terms they'll understand.

Others have described how their child stumbled upon their condoms or saw them taking birth control pills and asked what they were, leading to age-appropriate conversations about birth control.

If you haven't yet talked about birth control by the time your child is a teenager or hanging out seriously with a crush (whichever comes first), it's time to start. Kids learn the basics about driving years before they get behind a wheel; share information about condoms and contraception years before they need it too. This gives you time to lay the basic foundation (that people can become pregnant from penile-vaginal intercourse, that most people use contraception and there are different kinds; also, that STIs are common and there are ways to reduce risk). Then, over time, add more details. On average, teenagers start having oral sex around ages fourteen to seventeen and intercourse around ages sixteen to eighteen. Back each of these up by a couple of years to get a sense of when to start having more detailed talks.

Q. How can I help my teenager or young adult choose a birth control method that's right for them?

Most young people (especially college-bound teens) do not feel ready for a pregnancy. Although some are committed to abstinence, many others are sexually active (or hope to be soon) and want a highly effective method of preventing pregnancy. As a parent, you can help make your child aware of effective birth control options and either connect them with a doctor or nurse or let them know you support their choice to find a healthcare provider on their own. This is critical if your child lives or goes to school where abortion is illegal or severely restricted.

Many college students have been sexually active since high school but are terrified of their parents finding out, which keeps them from using effective forms of birth control. Some young people worry about disappointing their parents, while others worry about being kicked out of their home or shamed within their family or religious community. Young people need love, support, and guidance. With family support, they are better positioned to talk with a healthcare provider about their sexual health. Their provider can help them to choose a safe and highly effective birth control method that they can use consistently and correctly, as well as ask them some questions to check that they're not being abused or coerced into sex.

The most effective birth control methods are those that are not dependent on people's behavior or memory; they are provider-placed, such as IUD or implant, and offer years of protection. Yet, even the most effective birth control methods are not 100 percent perfect. Share that birth control methods fail sometimes, that doubling up on protection is helpful (adding withdrawal or condom use), and that they can come to you or another trusted adult for help and support if they have an unintended pregnancy. Also encourage them to discuss the possibility of pregnancy with their sexual partners, including what they would do if they become pregnant.

Q. What STI basics do teenagers need to know?

While I enjoy learning the nitty-gritty details about STIs, most people just want to know how to protect themselves and their partner(s). Here are some key messages to share:

- **Be open with one's doctor or nurse.** Telling one's provider about the kinds of sex they have (oral, vaginal, and/or anal sex) as well as the gender/sex of their sexual partner(s) can help their provider figure out which kinds of STI tests to offer and whether they need to check the throat, vagina, and/or rectum. How often people should get tested depends on their age, gender/sex, how many partners they have, gender/sex of their partner(s), and whether they have casual hookups or anonymous partners.
- **Most birth control methods don't protect against STIs.** Good news, though: condoms offer protection against several STIs and can be used in conjunction with other forms of contraception.
- **STIs are equal-opportunity infections.** While most people realize that STIs can be transmitted between males and females, as well as between two males, some don't realize that two females can transmit STIs to one another too. They can, through oral sex, vulva-to-vulva contact, and sharing sex toys.
- **Most STI testing is simple.** STIs can be tested for via urine screening or quick swabs of the throat, cervix, and/or rectum. HIV can be tested for through blood from a finger prick or from fluid from one's mouth.

- **Affordable STI testing often requires asking around.** Private doctor's offices may be expensive. Fortunately, some college health centers, family planning clinics, HIV organizations, and health departments offer sliding-scale pricing or community events with free testing.

- **There's no shame in having an STI.** About half of people will get an STI by the age of twenty-five, making it a fact of life for sexually active people and not a reflection of anyone's worth.

- **People who have an STI should let potential partners know before having sex.** Being open about one's STI status is caring and ethical. Also, in some states, if a person has HIV and doesn't disclose it to their partner, it may be considered a crime. Further, a person can get sued for monetary damages for failing to disclose a known STI to a partner. Let's normalize talking about STIs.

- **Follow-up STI testing may be needed.** People who are treated for bacterial STIs should ask their provider if they should return for repeat testing to make sure they've been cured of the infection. Some STIs are antibiotic resistant and may require additional treatment.

- **People can reduce their STI risk by abstaining from oral, vaginal, and anal sex or, if they're sexually active, by limiting their number of sexual partners.** For those who are sexually active, monogamy is least risky, especially if both partners have been tested. Those with multiple sex partners can reduce risk through consistent condom use and regular STI testing. HIV risk can be dramatically reduced through PrEP use.

- **Condoms should be used from start to finish.** Too many people start sex without a condom and add one midway or else they start with a condom on but take it off before ejaculation. These "partial use" scenarios increase risk of STIs (as well as pregnancy). Also, condoms should never be removed without telling one's partner—a practice called "stealthing" that, aside from being unethical, is also against some campus sexual misconduct policies and, in some places, against the law.

CONTRACEPTION AND MEANINGFUL CONSENT

Kristina and Susan once handled a case involving two college students, Alex and Madison, who, since their freshman year, had flirted with one another and hooked up on occasion. In their junior year, they decided to start having sex regularly. They agreed the sex was casual with no prospect of a dating relationship, and both were comfortable having sex without commitment. They talked about their sexual interests and agreed that they were comfortable engaging in sex without a condom because Madison was on the pill. After a few weeks of casual sex, Alex and Madison decided to move on from one another and stopped having sex.

Two weeks later, Madison learned that she had an STI. When she called Alex to let him know he should get tested, she learned that she wasn't Alex's first casual sex partner and that he had engaged in condomless sex with other women in the past. Madison felt furious and deeply misled by Alex. Although they had agreed not to use condoms, Madison said she only agreed to sex without a condom because she was under the impression that Alex hadn't had unprotected sex with anyone else (ever), which would have made him—in her eyes—a relatively low-risk partner, at least for some STIs. After learning that Alex had had unprotected sex with others, Madison now viewed the sex they'd had as nonconsensual, telling Alex that she would not have agreed to set condoms aside if she had known he had previously forgone condoms with others.

Feeling blindsided, Alex began to wonder whether he had properly obtained consent for sex. Was the validity of Madison's consent undermined by the fact that he hadn't disclosed to her that he had unprotected sex with other women in the past? How much information was Madison entitled to on topics she'd never asked about or said were important to her? It wasn't as if Alex lied to Madison or pressured her for sex without a condom; he just didn't share all the details of his sexual past. (Indeed, most people do not give all the details of their sexual pasts to others.)

As a college professor, I hear similar stories from students that highlight the importance of sexual partners making fully informed decisions together about condoms and other forms of contraception. One woman stayed after class to share that she was feeling stressed because one of her roommates had confided in her that she had lied to the guy she was sleeping with (a mutual friend) by telling him that she was taking birth control pills when she wasn't. They were using the withdrawal technique, and apparently the roommate didn't feel she was at high risk of pregnancy. However, withdrawal ("pulling out") doesn't always work. Moreover, it wasn't fair to this guy that the roommate was lying about being on the pill. This was not meaningful consent because the roommate was withholding key information from her sexual partner, and it was information that might have made him either not want to have sex with her or choose to use a condom instead of just pulling out. My student wondered whether she should tell their mutual friend that her roommate was lying to him.

Meaningful consent means that people put their cards on their table. They're open, transparent, and give their (potential) partner all the information they need to make an informed choice. Encourage your child to be honest with prospective partners and to ask the questions that they feel will give them the information they need. It's okay to ask about someone's sexual past, but that person also has the right not to answer if they feel it's no one else's business. And if you don't like the answer (or their silence), you don't have to have sex with that person. Everyone gets to make the choice that's right for them, their heart, their peace of mind, and their body.

"USE A CONDOM" ISN'T ENOUGH

Kristina and Susan have seen enough sexual misconduct cases that center around condom use that it suggests young people could benefit from more detailed information than "make sure you use a condom" (which is all that some teens hear from parents and schools). Some of these cases involve men refusing to wear condoms, either because they don't like how condoms feel or because they find it difficult to maintain their erection while using condoms. Others involve men who start out wearing a condom but then remove the condom during sex and re-insert their penis into their partner's vagina or anus without the condom. Each of these has implications for both consent and safety.

Fiona and Dante

College students Fiona and Dante struggled to figure out if they wanted to date. Part of that struggle was rooted in what they viewed as an initially "bad" (their words) sexual experience, in which Dante couldn't keep his erection during intercourse and it felt awkward for them both. Fiona and Dante initially decided not to hook up anymore, but after some months passed, they ended up trying to have intercourse again. Dante asked Fiona if she wanted to have sex and Fiona agreed. (So far so good in terms of clear verbal consent.) He got a condom and lubricant and they began intercourse. As Dante began to struggle with his erection, he asked Fiona to switch sexual positions multiple times, which she agreed to each time. But that didn't help his erection either.

Frustrated, Dante removed the condom and asked Fiona to perform oral sex on him, which helped him become erect again. Perhaps nervous about losing his erection yet again, Dante quickly resumed intercourse—this time without a condom. He didn't ask Fiona if it was okay to have sex without a condom and Fiona—although fearful about having sex without a condom and shocked that it was happening—didn't say anything. She didn't tell Dante "no" or "I'm not comfortable having sex without a condom." However, she also didn't expressly consent to sex without one. Instead, she lay there while Dante penetrated her. He seemed to take her lack of a "no" as consent—a bad idea, especially with a new sexual partner with whom no norms, routines, or boundaries have been established. Even regular partners should make sure to keep up their sexual communication.

In the days that followed, Fiona felt increasingly troubled by what had happened with Dante. She hadn't wanted to have sex with Dante without a condom nor had they discussed doing that. She wondered if it mattered whether Dante asked for consent to have sex without a condom since they had initially agreed to have intercourse with a condom. She also hadn't known how to navigate Dante's inability to maintain an erection and hadn't wanted to embarrass him. As Fiona sat with her feelings, she realized how violated she felt and filed a campus sexual misconduct complaint against Dante.

Please tell your teen or young adult that they should not jump into unprotected sex without clear consent from their partner; relying on their silence is not enough. There's too much at stake when it comes to pregnancy risk, STI risk, and making someone feel scared or violated. Before having sex without a condom, meaningful consent is needed—that is, consent obtained without pressure or coercion or making anyone feel rushed to decide. Just because someone has erection difficulties does not entitle them to have unprotected sex without consent. Their erection is not more important than their partner's comfort, safety, or ability to make their own choices about their own body and sexuality.

Sometimes two people agree to use withdrawal, but then one intentionally ejaculates inside their partner's vagina or anus. Or one person pressures their partner to have sex without a condom even though the partner doesn't want to. Usually, these situations are not filed as official reports but are discussed among partners ("You shouldn't have done that!") or confided about to close friends. That said, Kristina and Susan's experience is that they are sometimes filed as official sexual misconduct reports, especially given the risks involved when it comes to pregnancy and STIs. Even if you have to say it ten times, tell your child:

- **Don't remove a condom without clear communication and plenty of time for both you and the other person to think it through.** This is not the kind of decision to make on the fly.

- **Don't ejaculate in or on someone after telling them you won't.** Although mistakes happen, here we're referring to purposefully ejaculating somewhere without permission.
- **Never pressure someone into condomless sex.** Just because someone wants to have sex without a condom doesn't mean they're entitled to that. People should get to make this very big decision without feeling pressured or guilted into it.

Elijah and Luna

During their relationship, college students Elijah and Luna, who described themselves as having been in love with one another, had relied on condoms for birth control. Although neither wanted a pregnancy, Luna did not want to go on hormonal birth control because she was scared that her parents would discover that she was sexually active, and so they settled on using condoms. Yet, they both felt that sex with condoms didn't feel as pleasurable as sex without condoms. As their two-year anniversary approached, they decided to celebrate by taking a vacation together. Wanting their anniversary night to be romantic and sexy, Elijah and Luna ate dinner at a fancy restaurant and then had sex without a condom (they disagree on whether or not the condomless sex was consented to). Luna took emergency contraception (EC) the next morning. However, to her shock, she missed her period a couple of weeks later and discovered that she was pregnant. Luna opted to have an abortion, and the emotions surrounding their anniversary sex, unintended pregnancy, and decision to end the pregnancy led to their breakup. Luna then filed a campus sexual misconduct report against Elijah, alleging that she did not consent to their having unprotected sex. Elijah claimed that the reason they had EC with them was not as a backup but because they had planned to have condomless sex and use EC as pregnancy prevention. Cases like this one highlight the need for thoughtful conversations about pregnancy prevention, the value of using highly effective birth control, and that no one should be pressured to have unprotected sex. (They also highlight that EC is not perfect.)

When kids move away from home or head off to college, many families send along a first aid kit, self-care items (thermometer, nail clippers), and health insurance card, and store their healthcare provider's contact information in their child's phone. Try to anticipate your child's sexual health needs too. Ensure their HPV vaccine series has been completed, and consider packing the following items:

- **Safer sex products.** Include a variety of condoms (so they can find the ones that they and their partner like best) and water-based lubricant.
- **Pregnancy tests.** If there's any chance they'll have sex with other-sex partners, send along at least two at-home pregnancy tests. It's better to test early and understand all one's options than to wait.
- **Emergency contraception.** EC can help to reduce the risk of pregnancy up to five days after unprotected sex.
- **Birth control.** Talk about birth control options months before the big move, if possible, as it can take time to get an appointment with a healthcare provider and to find the birth control that works best for them in terms of side effects and ease of use.
- **Medications.** This includes preventive medications (like PrEP, if relevant to your child) and, if your child has a known STI, any medications they may need for prevention of flare-ups.
- **A sex book.** Choose a trustworthy LGBTQ+ inclusive book that addresses healthy relationships, condoms, birth control, STIs, genital anatomy, painful sex and how to prevent it, sexual pleasure, and orgasms.

4

Consent, Communication, and Care

Teenagers and young adults are in the early stages of an often exciting—albeit awkward and stressful—journey as they explore crushes, desire, intimacy, sexuality, and love. Along the way, there is bound to be heartbreak and rejection. Those who keep at it and grow their skills around communicating and connecting with others in vulnerable ways are also likely to experience pleasure and closeness with someone who becomes special to them.

Most parents want their kids to grow up and be able to create, if they so desire, intimate relationships that feel close, caring, pleasurable, and loving. Most young people want this for themselves too. They're eager to move past those early moments of trying to figure out how to kiss, when to reach for someone's hand, or how to let someone know about their feelings. Many teens and young adults want to be affectionate with someone who is special to them, whether that means cuddling with a crush, making out, or becoming sexually active with a partner. Some may be awakening to new kinds of pleasurable feelings in their bodies, which may feel surprising and sometimes overpowering thanks to hormonal changes. Sexuality is a life-long adventure!

Forming romantic relationships is a common part of adolescent and young adult development. Although there's risk involved, the risk goes both ways: There's a risk that things might not work out but there's also a chance they will. The possibility that one might find someone who they're attracted to, who they love being around, and who they can lean on keeps hope alive even in difficult times. A twenty-two-year-old in one of my research studies spoke to the power of forming close romantic relationships when he said, "We tend to think that family is 'supposed' to love us and knowing that a non-family member loves us makes us feel wanted. That gives our life meaning and a reason to keep going."

And yet, as much as young people want to explore romantically and/or sexually, they are acutely aware that they have no idea how to navigate this new terrain. If sexuality information from their school or family has been sparse, young people search for information wherever they can find it. Many kids ultimately learn about sex from magazines, locker room conversations, pornography, or the internet. Friends share information that they believe to be true.

Unfortunately, the information kids find through these sources is not always the kind that supports the development of caring relationships or mutually pleasurable sexual expression. Pornography often depicts sex in ways that are rough, aggressive, coercive, or that would be harmful, scary, or constitute sexual assault if enacted in real life. Too often, social media videos and online articles offer inaccurate and even harmful sex advice. This leaves young people with little fact-based or compassion-rich sexuality information to serve as a foundation for creating caring, intimate experiences. Even if you're confident that your child has not yet seen pornography or explicit social media videos, if their crush or romantic/sexual partner has gotten their sex education primarily from such sources, that may be enough to detour your child's early sexual experiences in potentially harmful ways.

In a college campus-representative survey, 41 percent of women, 11 percent of men, and about half of transgender and gender nonbinary students report having had at least one encounter in which an intimate experience that started out all right—kissing, making out, or having sex—ended up feeling frightening.[32] These students' stories are marked by sexual pressure, coercion, violence, and sexual assault.

Although teaching about consent is important, I hope we can agree that consent is the bare minimum expectation for partnered sex. As in most areas of life, people want more than just what's legally permissible. In hiring a sitter, parents don't settle for someone who meets only minimal criteria—as in, someone who will watch children without harming them. Rather, parents hire sitters who are trustworthy but also kind, creative, and fun. When looking for a place to live, people don't just want a home that squeaks by local safety ordinances. They want a home they love and feel they can be happy in, with features that feel important to them such as a large kitchen, natural sunlight, or a yard where their child can play. "Legal" is a starting place, offering necessary but rarely sufficient conditions for feeling good about one's choice. The same is true for sexual activities, whether they occur between teenagers or adults: Consent is important but it's not enough. We owe each other more. Imagine what kinds of pleasure and human connection might be possible if we raised the bar from mere consent to mutual pleasure and care.

In this chapter, you will find detailed information about sexual consent because even though it's the minimum expectation, it's still crucial to get right. Additionally, I've combed through hundreds of college students' stories to identify common problems they ran into in their first few years of making out and being sexually active to help you think through what you want to share with your child. The idea isn't to scare them but to offer them thoughtful guidance; imagine sharing a road map with your child, where you're encouraging them to enjoy their adventure but also to be careful of certain sharp turns and steep drop-offs.

DECISION-MAKING

One way to help young people do better with navigating consent, power dynamics, and others' feelings is by separating these issues from sex. Talk with your child about the everyday choices they and their friends make that have nothing to do with sex: If your teen has friends over and they want to watch a movie, but have different ideas about what movie to watch, how do they choose? Are decisions made together, or does one friend tend to call the shots while others give in? Do they flip a coin? Do they search for middle ground so that most people are happy? Paying attention to your own family dynamics, as well as how your child and their friends or special someone make day-to-day decisions together, creates opportunities to talk about communication, caring, and power. Look for opportunities to ask questions like:

- "It sounds like you and your friends have different ideas about what you're going to do when you hang out this weekend. How will you all decide?"
- "How do *you* feel about that decision?" and "How do you think *they* feel about that decision?"
- "How do you feel about the way you and your friends figured that out?" (This focuses on their process, not just the outcome.)
- "How do you and your friends make sure no one feels pressured to go along with something they're not comfortable doing?"
- "That sounds like a tough spot to be in. How will you work that out together?"

These questions encourage kids to consider how decisions get made and how those processes makes people feel. For families with more than one child, parents should pay attention to sibling power dynamics: Is the older or stronger sibling ruling the roost, or do all family members have a voice in the house? Introducing ideas of pressure and coercion in the context of decisions that have nothing to do with sex is one way to encourage them to think about power and how people use (and misuse) it. This builds an important foundation both for sexual communication and for important skills around empathy and compassion.

Further, naming what you see is a powerful tool; saying "I wonder if you felt pressured to go along with your friends" may open the door to hearing their perspective and to helping them imagine and plan for how they may be better able to push back against peer pressure in the future. Even young children may experience pressure, such as when a friend says they won't play with them unless they do a certain thing. Name this for them. Say, "It sounds like they're trying to control what you do. How do you feel about that?" At all ages, there are opportunities to talk about both power and care. Young people are smart and, with practice, they become skilled at noticing if someone is pressuring another person to do something. They can also spot when they're the ones doing the pressuring and can learn to stop themselves and change how they're acting toward their friend, classmate, family member, or person they're dating.

PLANNING AHEAD

Humans have a unique capacity to plan ahead and to imagine what they might do in certain situations. When children are young, parents prepare them for the first day of school by letting them know that, when they arrive at their classroom, they will be shown to their cubby or desk and then put away their backpack or school supplies. For teens and young adults, planning looks different, but the strategy is the same: One imagines what might happen and prepares for what they will do, need, or say. If a teenager wants to go to a party but doesn't want to give in to pressure to drink alcohol, they can rehearse how they will respond when someone offers them a beer. If a person expects to have sex, they can plan ahead by bringing condoms and/or meeting in advance with a healthcare provider to talk through birth control options. If a young adult is meeting up with a stranger they met through a dating app, they can imagine what they will say if the person asks them to leave their public meeting spot and go back to their place.

It also helps kids to hear from their parents, in specific terms, what is and is not okay. You may feel like you don't or shouldn't need to say these things to your child. Yet, the fact that so many young people have had scary sexual experiences suggests that all parents should be having these conversations with their children—even if you feel certain that your child would never hurt a soul. These conversations may also help your child to spot red flags at earlier stages of getting to know someone. Further, they are opportunities to help your child imagine scenarios and create mental plans about what they will do or say should certain situations arise.

AFFIRMATIVE CONSENT

Many college campus policies require affirmative consent for sex. Often referred to as "yes means yes," affirmative consent generally requires that people demonstrate a resounding yes to sexual activity at each step of a sexual encounter. This can (usually) be done either verbally (saying "yes") or nonverbally (such as a clear nodding of the head), but it must be clear, voluntary, and not pressured or coerced. Consent obtained through coercion is not valid consent. Kristina and Susan often liken affirmative consent to the children's game "Mother May I?" where, instead of asking "May I take two steps?" young people are expected to ask if they can kiss, take one another's clothes off, or have oral sex.

Affirmative consent policies sound reasonable; after all, a yes to one thing (such as oral sex) does not mean a yes to anything else (such as vaginal sex or anal sex). However, given how sexual activity tends to unfold in real life, particularly with young people who are new to sex, affirmative consent policies can present challenges. Studies consistently find that most young people do not use (nor do they expect their partners to use) explicit verbal consent for most kinds of sexual activities, including kissing, breast touching, genital touching, and oral sex.[33] They tend to use implicit verbal communication (e.g., "Should I get a condom?" instead of asking "Do you

The Sexual Consent Spectrum

The following are all ways that people may communicate sexual consent, from the clearest ("Explicit verbal consent") to the least clear ("No response," which may mean that it's all right with a person, but it could also mean that a person is feeling pressured, coerced, or too scared to say no). Especially with newer partners, it's safer and wiser to use verbal communication or other clear forms of consent.

Most Clear ↑

Explicit verbal consent
"Do you want to have sex?"

Implicit verbal consent
"Should I get a condom?"

Explicit nonverbal consent
Person gets a condom.

Implicit nonverbal consent
Person takes off their clothes.

No response
Person does not resist or say no.

↓ Least clear

want to have intercourse?") or else just keep things moving forward (kissing, then breast/chest touching, then genital touching, and so on) unless someone says no or pushes the other person away. Students often tell Kristina and Susan that they believed they had consent simply from the removal of clothing and not from any conversation; make sure your child knows that taking someone's clothes off, and them not resisting, isn't the same as clear consent. The person whose clothes are being removed may be feeling scared or unsure about what to do.

Although this lack of communication is fine for some people at times, it doesn't work for everyone. People tend to talk about sex in vague, coded ways, and that's when they talk about it at all. Many adults avoid talking directly about sex, too, instead developing their own coded ways of inviting their partner to have sex—perhaps you or your partner have said something like "The kids are out and we have the house to ourselves" before, without actually saying anything about sex. This can work in long-term relationships in which people have developed a shared meaning (and often shared sexual routines). However, being vague and nonspecific presents problems for newer sexual partners. Learning to talk clearly about sex is so important. Doing so in a culture of silence and shame is no easy task, but sex tends to go better—and consent is clearer—when people use their words.

WHAT IT MEANS TO CONSENT

Too often, young people are simply told "Make sure you get consent" or "No means no" without additional detail. At its most basic, consent needs to be freely given and clearly communicated, and the people involved must be conscious—not asleep or incapacitated by alcohol or drugs. But school policies may, as described earlier, require more than that. If your child's school requires verbal consent for sexual activity, then be clear with your child about how important it will be for them and their friends to use words when they communicate about making out or having sex. They need to understand, in no uncertain terms, that it may not be enough to just take off each other's clothes and proceed to sexual activities (no matter how eager everyone involved seems). Instead, they would be wise to use words like "Would you like to have sex?" and then wait to hear the other person say "Yes" (not just nod their head). Likewise, consent should ideally be given for each new type of sex—especially with newer partners who haven't established a regular routine together. Just because a person asks and receives consent for oral sex doesn't mean that they have consent for intercourse.

While making out or having sex, verbal consent communications may involve one person asking if they can go down on their partner or get a condom and the other person saying "Yes" or "Mmm-hmmmm" or "I'd like that." Moaning does not constitute consent, nor does it necessarily mean that the other person is enjoying sex. While this may seem obvious to you as an adult with years of experience, it's not obvious to many young people; Kristina and Susan have seen many cases where young men misinterpreted moaning to mean consent, making their partner feel violated and landing themselves in trouble. Although moaning often reflects pleasure, moaning can also reflect discomfort or pain, including vaginal pain, anal pain, or pelvic pain (such as from endometriosis). People also sometimes moan to get their partner to stop sex. That may seem counterintuitive. Yet, many young people (and women in particular) find it difficult to experience orgasm and/or feel pressured by their partner to have an orgasm, and so they pretend to have one either to make their partner happy or because they don't want to be having sex any longer and just want their partner to finish and be done.

Relying on one's partner just going along with what's happening is an unhelpful, and insufficient, method of discerning consent. And again—consent is the bare minimum. The goal is sex that's enjoyable for both partners, not just sex that doesn't harm people or get them in trouble. With my college students, I often talk about how people can co-create sex that is wanted, pleasurable, and feels good for each partner. We discuss the importance of choosing partners who care about them as human beings, and of being thoughtful about their own sexual choices. Just because someone consents to sex does not mean it will feel good to them either in the moment or the next day. If a person's ex wants them to get back together, they may initiate sex as a way of reconnecting. But that doesn't mean that having sex is good for that person's heart, soul, or well-being. It may cause heartache and confusion. So, there's consent and then there's being a caring human being who works toward good things for other people, especially when they are entrusted with other people's bodies and/or hearts.

WAS IT ASSAULT?

Sixteen-year-old Mia came to see Kristina and Susan because she was worried she had done something wrong and could be kicked out of school or worse. Weeks earlier, Mia had engaged in what she believed was a consensual sexual experience with one of her closest friends, Lizzie, one evening after drinking some wine from Mia's parents' liquor cabinet. Neither one was incapacitated, though certainly the wine had lessened their inhibitions. Mia and Lizzie started to engage in touching, kissing, and, eventually, oral sex. To Mia, the experience was an exploration of whether she was sexually attracted to girls generally or to Lizzie more specifically. And even though both young women had felt fine about their sexual exploration, high school rumors can be harsh: in the following days, rumors swirled through their high school, and students began calling Mia a rapist because they had heard that Mia had offered Lizzie alcohol during their sexual encounter.

Mia wanted legal advice, but she also wanted to hear the opinion of lawyers about whether she had indeed assaulted one of her best friends, someone she cared about deeply. Clearly, raiding her parents' liquor cabinet was wrong. But was their sexual experience nonconsensual simply because they had been drinking? Mia felt confused, regretful, and ashamed. What had felt like a consensual experience to both her and Lizzie at the time of the actual event had morphed into something negative and shameful by the time news of it made its way through their school. Kristina and Susan assured Mia that she was not a rapist by any stretch of the imagination. Mia needed that reassurance because of her confusion around the meaning of consent. Kristina and Susan explained that drinking does not negate consent if both people have the ability to understand who they are, where they are, and what is going on. And, in this case, both people had perceived their exploration positively until the rumors spread.

Mia's experience highlights some of the difficulties understanding consent and sexual assault among students. Young people often ask if sex is nonconsensual if they or their partner consumed any amount of alcohol.

They ask: How drunk is incapacitated versus just intoxicated? How can you tell the difference? Also, in Mia's case the term *rape* hadn't even occurred to her until some of their friends insinuated that Lizzie was raped because she drank some wine before agreeing to let Mia perform oral sex on her. Kristina and Susan have seen many sexual misconduct and assault cases where the rumor mill turned a formative sexual experience into a scandal. Judgment by peers, most of whom also have very little sexual experience or life experience, is not only hurtful but potentially harmful, especially if those peers are making serious accusations. Many of us probably remember being part of some high school drama that led to whispers and rumors. That still happens today, only it's often amplified through social media and anonymous online posts.

CARE, COMMUNICATION, AND DECENCY

Consent can get even more confusing when it involves dating relationships. Kristina and Susan have seen many cases where, after a couple breaks up, one person files a sexual misconduct or sexual assault complaint discussing an event that might have occurred weeks, months, or even years, earlier in the relationship. Often, young people don't realize how important it can be to keep checking in with their partner to make sure that the sexual activities in which they're engaging are wanted and consensual. Even if two people have sex with one another numerous times, it does not mean that they want to keep having sex. People fall out of love or lust. They lose interest. Sometimes people realize that they no longer enjoy certain kinds of sex that used to bring them pleasure—or that they once went along with because they didn't know how to decline or say "not like that." People change their hearts and their minds for any number of reasons.

Young people need to make sure that their partner is truly interested in being sexual together. The clearest way is to use words ("Would you like to have sex?" or "Can I go down on you?" or "How about we just cuddle tonight?"). But we live in the real world and know, from both personal and professional experience, that most people don't ask questions every time they have sex, and certainly not for every aspect of sex. That said, you can still encourage your child to use words for sexual communication (especially with newer partners) and to check in with their partner from time to time.

Another way to help your child navigate sex in ways that are transparent and consensual is to encourage your child to approach hooking up and sexual situations with care, kindness, and human decency. Tell them:

- They shouldn't pretend to love someone just to have sex with them.
- They shouldn't rush sex. It's not their job to "take things to the next level" or "move the ball forward," especially with someone who seems unsure.
- If someone only wants a friends-with-benefits situation (they don't want to date or be in a relationship), they should clearly communicate that. They can say, "I'm only interested in hooking up; I'm not interested in anything romantic or exclusive."
- If they are looking to date or be in a relationship, they need to say that too—even if it means losing someone who only wants casual hookups. Here's how: "To be clear, I like you and I'm interested in dating you; I'm not into just hooking up or something casual, which would be too hard on me and hurt my feelings. So please, let's only do this if you share those feelings."
- Even if they and their partner decide to be in an open relationship (meaning one or both of them can be sexual with others), that doesn't mean their partner will be okay with them sleeping with that partner's best friend, ex-boyfriend/girlfriend, roommate, fraternity brother, or sorority sister. There are some lines that are too sensitive to cross. They should tread carefully and talk it through with their partner.

As discussed earlier, there are many ways for parents to communicate these and other ideas about sex and relationships. Watching television or movies alongside your child will yield many opportunities to talk about caring approaches to sex as well as sexual consent and communication. If a character in a show pretends to want an exclusive relationship just so they can have sex with someone, you might say, "Even though the sex was technically consensual, because one person asked if they could have sex and the other said yes, it didn't seem kind or caring because the guy lied about wanting a relationship just to get sex. He misrepresented his intentions and that's not how people deserve to be treated. What do you think?"

COMMUNICATION ROADBLOCKS

Clear communication is important for establishing consent for anything from kissing to intercourse; it's also helpful for creating sex that feels good to people. Yet, many young people of all ages avoid talking about sex for various reasons including:

- **Embarrassment or shame.** For some people, their religion, culture, family, or schools have been shaming about sex. Many people recall asking a parent, grandparent, or teacher about something to do with penises, vaginas, or sex, only to be told not to talk about that or "that's dirty." People who feel ashamed to talk about sex sometimes find it difficult to tell someone that they're not ready for or interested in a certain kind of sex.

- **Lack of experience.** In one study, about 60 percent of eighteen- to twenty-four-year-old women said that discomfort talking about sex kept them from communicating with their partner. In contrast, only 29 percent of twenty-five- to twenty-nine-year-old women felt that way, demonstrating how much change happens during young adulthood.[34] If a person has never before said the word *condom* out loud, they may be unlikely to ask "Do you have a condom?" or say "I'm not comfortable having sex unless we use a condom." As a parent, you can model mature conversations about sex and gender topics to give your child practice well before they become sexually active.

- **Fear of ruining the moment.** Some people worry they'll ruin the mood by talking about sex. Yet, talking helps make sure that people are on the same page and feel safe, comfortable, and completely into it (whatever "it" is). Some people talk ahead of time—sharing whether they're ready for intercourse and, if not, what might help them feel ready one day. This might include being exclusive, getting STI/HIV testing, using condoms or other forms of birth control, or feeling in love. Some people want to be engaged or married before having sex. Using words helps to share and understand one another's needs.

- **Feeling uncertain about the words themselves.** Although sensational forms of sex often seem ever-present in the media, sexuality education remains rare. Thus, many people have never heard, let alone said out loud, words like *clitoris*. They aren't sure how to pronounce it and shy away from saying it. (If you're also unsure, most sex educators say "CLIT-or-iss" but some people say "cli-TOHR-iss" and that's okay too.) Because no one wants to seem clueless about sex, some people stay silent rather than risk seeming inexperienced. If your own uncertainty about saying sex words out loud is getting in the way of talking with your child, try watching some sex education videos yourself (see **Resources**).

- **Exposure to sex myths.** We are inundated with sex myths. Some people have been raised to believe that "good girls" aren't supposed to even think about sex, let alone ask for sex. There are also harmful myths that men must always want sex and have sex whenever the opportunity presents itself—even if that means with a drunk person who is coming on to them (not okay). These are important myths for parents to counter.

While these are common reasons young people find it difficult to talk about sex, they don't tell the whole story. There are other reasons—some quite difficult—that complicate sexual communication and consent. For example:

- **An inability to move.** When faced with fear, some people fight back or try to escape ("fight or flight"). Others get stuck in what's called "fight or flight on hold," which is when their body freezes. This is more common for people who suffer from post-traumatic stress disorder stemming from having been physically or sexually assaulted or having lost a loved one. But anyone can freeze up. And the fact that some people freeze in response to feeling sexually threatened is one reason that it's important to never assume a person is okay with sex just because they don't resist or say no. If a partner is not participating with any enthusiasm, regardless of previous consent, it's important to check in and ask the person if the sex should stop. If the other person looks like they're falling asleep or passing out or more drunk than it initially seemed, they should stop sex immediately.

- **Fears about a partner hurting them.** Some people—especially women—who want to get out of a sexual situation feel afraid that their partner will be angry, aggressive, or violent if they try to end things. Consequently, they may not speak up or push back, even when asked or made to do something sexual that they don't like. This is especially true for people who have grown up witnessing domestic violence. To help your child stay safe, teach them to identify controlling and/or abusive characteristics in others. Because intimate partner violence is prevalent, and it can take an average of seven tries to leave an abusive situation,[35] parents can be a steady source of love and support so that their child isn't as isolated as an abusive partner might want them to be.

- **Abuse or trauma.** Figuring out one's boundaries is a normal part of sexual exploration, and I've heard from many students who, while making out or being sexual with someone, came to a place where they didn't want to go any further. Unfortunately, it's also ripe for sexual conflict, with one partner wanting to take things farther and the other wanting to stop. Sometimes the person who wants to keep going exerts sexual pressure or coercion, saying, "We've gone this far, why not keep going?" Other times, the person continues with various sex acts even after hearing the word no. People who are being sexually assaulted may stop saying "no" because they feel resigned to what is happening, in shock about what has already happened, or retraumatized from prior experiences. Those with histories of molestation or assault may feel that saying "no" or "stop" yet again is pointless. Because this happens so commonly, I cannot say it enough: Parents need to tell their children of all genders that, if someone says "no," respect it the first time. Tell them that "no" means stop; it does not mean try harder.

While many long-term couples eventually fall into rhythms and routines where they don't say much before or during sex, familiarity and trust take time to build. Encourage your teen or young adult to clearly communicate when they are making out and being sexual with one another, especially with newer partners.

MEANINGFUL CONSENT

Sometimes people consent to sex but then later receive information that leaves them feeling misled about the surrounding circumstances, causing them to reevaluate whether that consent was coerced. To be able to give meaningful consent to sex, people need the most pertinent information that might affect their decision-making, such as whether the other person is:

- Of legal age to consent to have sex;
- Under the influence of drugs or alcohol;
- In a relationship or having sex with other people;
- Into something casual or interested in dating;
- Positive for any STIs, and how recently they were tested;
- Using birth control and, if so, what kind (for those with an other-sex partner).

People may hide information from someone they're attracted to, fearing that the person they like will reject them if they find out that they have an STI, they have other partner(s), or they are not of legal age to consent to sex.

Even so, be clear with your child that these are key pieces of information that they *must* share with potential partners.

Another way to help your child is to remind them how important it is to show kindness, even in the face of hearing difficult information. If your child is on the receiving end of such information, they can thank the person for being honest with them. If the person is too young to consent to sex, they need to part ways ("I'm sorry, I think you're great but we can't legally have sex and I don't want to hurt you or get into trouble"). If the person has an STI, then they can learn about the STI together and see if they can find a way forward that feels comfortable to each partner. As we saw in Chapter 3, some STIs are curable and others can be treated in ways that reduce the risk of transmission.

THE TROUBLE WITH TEXTS

Given how much of young people's social lives takes place online, it is not surprising that they often use texts and social media to talk with their crushes, relationship partners, and potential hookup partners about their sexual desires. Many parents find it difficult to believe that their shy, school-oriented, sixteen-year-old would go into such explicit detail about their sexual fantasies over text, but it's not unusual. For many young people, it's easier to text about sex than to talk about it face-to-face. It's difficult for many adults to have vulnerable conversations about sex with their spouses of decades. Why would we expect this to be any easier for young people, who are brand-new to sex?

Too often, text exchanges play a pivotal role in sexual miscommunication. Sometimes people text or message about what they're into sexually, but when they get together in person, one of them takes the texts literally and starts to act out what was described without further discussion. Kids need to hear—loud and clear—that those texts do not necessarily reflect genuine interest in doing sexual things in real life, nor do they necessarily constitute consent. What matters most is what people decide together in the moment.

This means that if two people are texting—even in great, steamy detail—about kissing one another and then having intercourse, they should still talk about it when they meet up. Is that still something they're interested in doing? If so, what do they need to create sex that feels safe and pleasurable to them? Condoms? Birth control? A conversation about each other's STI status?

Let your child know that texting may be part of sexual communication but it shouldn't be all of it (just as giving your child an age-appropriate book shouldn't substitute for in-person sex talks). Also, if they are just having fun and sharing fantasies over text, encourage them to say—as part of the text exchange—something that makes it clear that this is just for fun and not necessarily what they're ready to do in real life. ("To be clear, this is just fantasy—not ready to do this in person.") Otherwise, the other person may take cues from their texts, which may lead to misunderstandings and even assault.

SEXUAL PRESSURE AND COMPLIANCE

Another important point to share with your child is that just because someone agrees to something may not mean it is consensual; the other person may have felt pressured to give in. *Sexual compliance* is a term that scientists use for giving in to a sexual experience that a person doesn't truly want. All too often, sexual compliance is normalized within families and cultures. This is especially true for girls and young women, who are frequently told "don't rock the boat" whether at school, at home, or in relationships.

Even though many young women today feel empowered to explore their bodies, to masturbate, and to experience sex as pleasurable and orgasmic, I still hear from many teenage girls and young women (though certainly not girls and women exclusively) who seem to be going along with sex rather than actively creating a joyful sex life with their partner. In anticipation of their first vaginal intercourse, many young women ask their friends or search the internet for tips on "how to make sex not hurt" instead of how to make sex feel good. This is a subtle difference, but it's an important one.

Kristina, Susan, and I also still hear stories about men who, when refused intercourse, ask their partner to "at least" give them a blow job. They feel entitled asking for it, and some partners feel obliged to go along with it. This is where seemingly offhand comments like "What, are you going to leave me with blue balls?" are not just crass but strategic, as they're about guilting or pressuring someone into doing something sexual they don't want to do. Similarly, sexual pressure can involve whining or repeatedly asks for sex with a "C'mon, can't we?"

Sexual pressure comes in various forms. Some students have described situations where a person they were hooking up with only told them they had an STI after they had been making out for a while, had built up arousal, and were about to start intercourse. On one hand, it's good that the person was forthcoming about having an STI before intercourse began. On the other hand, sharing one's STI status only when their partner is highly aroused and unlikely to be thinking logically isn't fair. It doesn't give the other person enough time to think things through clearly. Others have described feeling pressured in the midst of sex when a partner suddenly removes a condom and asks, "Just for a minute can we try it without a condom? I won't come inside you." This is not sufficient time for such a big decision and is yet another form of sexual pressure.

If someone feels pressured, coerced, afraid, or otherwise does not feel that they can safely refuse, that isn't true consent, because it isn't an equal playing field. Sexual pressure is something a person does to get what they want, not to create a mutually pleasurable experience. Further, sex that is pressured or coerced may be considered sexual misconduct or sexual assault.

Aiden and Jack

Kristina and Susan worked on a campus sexual misconduct case that involved two young men whose relationship had recently ended. Aidan was a popular, energetic student who was shocked to learn that his ex-boyfriend, Jack, who was more of an introvert, said that throughout their relationship he had felt pressured by Aidan to bottom during anal sex. From Aidan's perspective, he felt that the person who was the bottom (i.e., the recipient of anal sex) often felt more vulnerable and less pleasured than the partner who was the top, but that feeling vulnerable wasn't the same as being pressured or coerced. As the case unfolded, it turned out that both young men felt that bottoming was painful and neither one thought it was as fun or as pleasurable as topping. However, Jack shared that he had long felt like he was giving in to something he didn't enjoy whenever he let Aidan top.

The sexual dynamics between Aidan and Jack were complicated, and neither partner felt respected nor understood by the other. Aidan felt that Jack was insecure about sexual experimentation. Jack experienced the relationship as one of lack of respect and pressure. Jack also reported feeling belittled by Aidan, which likely contributed to him giving in to pressure. Both partners were suffering and could not navigate the relationship. Their sexual difficulties were influenced by a lack of sexual communication and likely by sexual incompatibility. Two men who both want to be tops can sometimes make a relationship work, especially if they find other kinds of sex they both enjoy or if they have an open relationship that involves permission to be sexual with others. But it's complicated. Ultimately, even though Aidan and Jack didn't feel right for one another, they learned about sexual communication, meaningful consent, and more about expressing their desires and boundaries.

PEOPLE CAN CHANGE THEIR MINDS

Be clear with your child that they or a partner can change their mind about intimacy and sex at any point. Someone might start to move toward vaginal sex only to remember that they forgot to take their birth control pill two days in a row. Or they might agree to vaginal or anal intercourse only to find that their partner's penis is bigger than they're comfortable accepting into their body. Might it be disappointing for one or both people to change their mind? Sure. But disappointment is part of life. What's important is that the person who no longer wants to do the intimate or sexual thing clearly communicates their choice to stop and that the person hearing it stops immediately. One can say:

- "I'm not comfortable doing this."
- "I've changed my mind."
- "I'm not ready."
- "I think I'm just going to go home."
- "This doesn't feel right."
- "That hurts."
- "Can you please get off me?"
- "I don't feel well."
- "I'm attracted to you but not comfortable with _____."

Or they just might say "stop." Women sometimes feel afraid to stop a sexual situation, especially if they initiated it, for fear of being called a tease or being forced into sex anyway. Men sometimes feel afraid to stop sex because stereotypes suggest men are supposed to always want and be ready for sex. No matter what gender a person is, their partner needs to respect when they say anything even remotely close to "stop" or indicate that they have changed their mind or are too tired and just want to go to sleep.

One of the most common scary sexual situations that people describe is when a person has consented to sex and then tries to stop it, only to find that their partner does not stop. They may say "stop" or "that hurts" and find that their partner tells them to be quiet, that they're ruining the mood, or to ignore them until they've finished. None of these are okay. Alice, a twenty-year-old college junior, described how her ex-boyfriend would regularly persist with sex even after she told him to stop:

There would be times we'd be having sex and it would hurt a lot. Like, I thought I tore something and bleeding was common, and I'd be, like, oh my God, stop. Like, it really, really hurts. And [my boyfriend] would be like, "I'm almost done." So I didn't even really let it show how much it bothered me. 'Cause I was like, all right, whatever, it'll just be like another thirty seconds, but it was really fucked up. Like it was not supposed to happen like that.

Their differences in size (her body was small and she described him as much larger) made her feel vulnerable and scared to resist any more than she had already tried. Given how common this scenario is, it is critical for parents to talk about the importance of being a caring partner who listens and stops whenever they are asked to stop, or whenever their partner seems sad, upset, or no longer having fun. At all times, no means no and stop means stop.

These situations are made more complicated by the fact that the person subjected to the consent violation (the one who said "stop" but whose partner persisted) sometimes doubts themselves. In reflecting on her experiences, Alice described how she would sometimes wonder, "Maybe it was me who was, like, not making it serious enough or, like, not establishing that boundary. But obviously if someone says to stop, you stop. Like, that's the whole basis of consent."

What Do I Say?

How to Share What Not to Do

Perhaps you've seen examples of sexual assault prevention messages passed around on the internet where advice like "Don't walk alone at night" has been crossed out and substituted with statements like "Don't rape people." This challenges the idea that it's the victim's responsibility to prevent their own assault and instead turns the focus on the actions of potential perpetrators. I've thought about this more often since getting to know Kristina and Susan and hearing about their cases—especially combined with findings from my team's research studies, in which clear patterns of problematic behavior emerge. Both parents and educators can and should do more to engage young people in conversations about how to avoid doing things that might make sex feel scary, coercive, or intimidating, or like others don't have a choice about what's happening. For example, you can tell your teen or young adult:

- **Do not isolate people, especially under false pretenses.** Too many sexual assault stories begin with a person being led somewhere isolated. They often involve a guy isolating a girl somewhere where she is acutely aware of how alone she is. Sometimes he invites her to his house to watch a movie only for her to arrive and find his parents aren't home. Other times, it's to take what seems like a romantic walk across campus or through a neighborhood, only to take a turn and wind up in an empty wooded area. While hooking up in a hidden place may seem exciting, it can also be scary. Some so-called pickup-artist books and websites advise men to get women away from their "pack" of friends so that they can make their move, even using analogies of predators hunting prey on the savannah. This is bad advice; tell your child not to follow it. Instead, share that an important part of being romantically or sexually involved with someone is that both people feel safe, comfortable, and able to make the choices that feel right to them.

- **Be thoughtful about differences in strength and size.** Many people, due to having a smaller body size or being with a partner who is bigger or stronger, are aware that they could easily be overpowered by their partner. People who are big, strong, and/or athletic should be caring and compassionate about these differences. Especially to someone new they're dating or hanging out with, they could say, "I know I'm bigger than you, and I want to make sure you always feel comfortable around me. If at any time you want to pause or stop or leave, just let me know. I will respect that."

- **Let people leave.** If someone wants to leave, let them leave—even if it's in the middle of making out or having sex. This goes back to body sovereignty and making sure people get to do what they want with their own body. Too often, people feel stuck or are physically restrained from getting up or leaving. Kristina and Susan have shared that in criminal cases of rape, it is not unusual that a kidnapping charge is also filed when one person doesn't allow the other to leave the room. Although we cannot blame everything on porn, many young people (and especially young men) describe learning how to have sex from watching it, and some of what they learn involves restraining a partner. People should always be free to leave, so tell them not to lock the door for privacy unless both people agree on that; to avoid standing between someone and the door; and never to restrain a partner without their clear, explicit, and enthusiastic consent. Say, "Do not hold their arms above their head. Do not pin them down by their wrists. Do not tie them up" (unless, of course, someone specifically asks for and clearly consents to that kind of sex).

- **Do not hold a person's head down during oral sex without clear, explicit, and enthusiastic consent.** Yes, this is an explicit conversation to have with one's own teenager or young adult but say it anyway; if you can say "Use a condom" you can say "Don't hold anyone's head down." For some people, having their head held down feels like they're being made to perform oral sex and that stopping or leaving is not an option.

We'd all like to think that our child would never hurt a soul and yet, clearly, many people's children do—sometimes unintentionally. Given the high rate of sexual assault (not to mention scary sexual situations that may not technically rise to the level of assault, but that are still harmful), it's a good idea for parents to be proactive with these conversations.

The Consequences Are Real

Make sure your child understands that there are real (and very serious) consequences for campus sexual misconduct as well as for criminal convictions of sexual assault. Sharing this information with your kid isn't a scare tactic; they should understand the severity of potential repercussions.

The worst outcome is the harm to another human being, which cannot be undone. Additionally, people who are found responsible for campus sexual misconduct may be suspended from school, expelled from school, or have their degree taken away (even after having completed the educational requirements of the institution). In criminal proceedings, people may go to jail or find themselves on a sex offender registry for many years, which has implications for where they can live, who they can have contact with, and what kinds of jobs may be open to them.

MOST SEXUAL ASSAULTS ARE NEVER REPORTED

More than 90 percent of college sexual assaults are never reported to authorities, whether to campus officials or police.[36] Most often, if a person tells anyone at all, it's a close friend.[37] Less often, students tell a family member. However, one study found that about 20 percent of women and about one quarter of men who experienced nonconsensual sex didn't tell anyone at all—not even a healthcare provider or crisis line.

There are many reasons for this. Some people tell themselves that what happened to them "wasn't that bad." Others worry they won't be believed. As one young woman who experienced a horrific sexual assault as a teenager said to me, "If I had had an adult in my life who I could have talked to, and I was absolutely sure that they wouldn't call me a liar or that they would believe me, maybe I would've spoken about it."

Also, young people who aren't yet out to their family or friends as LGBTQ+ but who were assaulted by someone of their own gender/sex—and perhaps met that person through an LGBTQ+ social event or hookup app—may fear being outed. Women and LGBTQ+ survivors often don't want to have to tell and retell their traumatic experiences to police officers and others in the judicial system, most of whom are straight men. Teenagers and young adults from religious or culturally conservative homes often say they don't tell family or report their assaults for fear of being judged or kicked out of their home, especially if leading up to the assault they did something they worry they'll be blamed for, such as having drunk alcohol, used a hookup app, or gone to someone's dorm room or apartment. Again, the best way to support your child is to create a warm, loving relationship with them. Say, "I will always love you and if you need help, I want you to feel like you can come to me."

IF YOUR CHILD HAS BEEN SEXUALLY ASSAULTED

If your child shares that they have been sexually assaulted, the most important thing you can do is to love and support them. Saying "I believe you" and "It's not your fault" and "I'm sorry this happened to you" go a long way. This is not a time to ask why, such as why they were wearing a certain outfit or drinking alcohol or at a party alone.

If the sexual assault just occurred, and if your child is open to this, you may want to suggest that they have a sexual assault response team medical examination (a SART exam). The healthcare providers who conduct these exams have special training in working with sexual assault survivors. The exams do, however, take a long time to conduct and can feel very personal, as they involve a close inspection of the entire body as well as photographs of any affected areas that may have scratches, bruises, bite marks, or other injuries. This is not to deter anyone from a SART exam; they are important forms of clinical care and documentation. However, some students have shared that they wish they had known what was involved prior to the exam. If your child is open to having a SART exam, it does not lock them into having to continue with official reports or speaking to police. And if they want you or a friend or other family member there for support, they can ask for that. Whenever possible, give your child a say over what is happening. A person who has been sexually assaulted or raped has experienced a loss of control over their own body. Being allowed to make choices about their own body—such as whether or not to take a shower, have a SART exam, or file a report—is vital. If your child chooses to have a SART examination, it's best to do so immediately, without changing clothing or showering, so that the nurse can collect any available evidence.

Sexual abuse and assault are epidemics. Even though we know this, many parents feel shocked, angry, and guilty when they learn their own child has been harmed. These are common reactions, even when there is nothing one could have done to prevent the assault. If you need support processing what happened to your child, please know that calling a crisis line is available for family members too—not just the survivor.

Finally, keep in mind that people who have experienced sexual trauma can and usually do go on to have fulfilling relationships and satisfying sex lives. Find opportunities to share this message more than once, especially if you know your child has been sexually abused or assaulted (but share this information even if you have no reason to believe they've been assaulted, just in case). Sexual harm is common and what's worse is that many people walk away feeling like they are damaged goods. Yet, most people—whether with the help and support of their own mind/body healing, loving friends or partners, and/or a professional—do find that they can move on, excel in school and at work, and create joyful, satisfying, and exciting sexual lives for themselves.

Collective Wisdom

Sexual communication and consent are the basis for both safe and pleasurable sex. Learning to talk about sex takes time and practice. Some recommendations to pass along to your child:

1. **For at least the first ten times a person has sex with a new partner, they should use explicit verbal consent.** This means they should use words rather than head nods or other nonverbal cues, even if it seems awkward. Ten is not a magic number, but sometimes having a guideline in mind can help. Also, talking about sex—such as asking "Do you want to have sex?"—gets easier with practice.

2. **Verbal consent is also wise any time something new is added.** For example, if a couple has been having oral sex together for a while, they should talk before moving on to vaginal or anal intercourse. They shouldn't assume that silence means "yes."

3. **If a person does not want to do something sexual, a verbal refusal is the clearest way to communicate that.** A verbal refusal also helps to establish lack of consent, if it comes to that. Examples are "No," "I'm not ready for intercourse," and "I'm attracted to you, but I don't want to have sex tonight."

4. **Blue balls never killed anyone.** Having blood flow gather in the genitals can sometimes hurt, but it does resolve with time and distraction. Also, people who are highly aroused can masturbate on their own for relief. Tell your teen that if someone has already declined sex, that person should not be asked to watch or assist the other person in masturbating, which is one strategy people use to keep others engaged in a sexual interaction with them and then escalate it to oral sex or intercourse. Their "no" must be respected.

5. **When in doubt, focus on being a compassionate, caring human being.** If someone says "Stop" or "That hurts," then stop immediately. If someone says they're not feeling well or they're still in pain from a recent illness or medical procedure, they shouldn't be pressured into sex—no matter how aroused one feels. Compassion is key.

6. **Be prepared.** Encourage your child to always have a charged cell phone, some money or a credit card, and the ability to call you, a friend, or a ride service if they need to leave an unsafe situation. Some families have a "no questions asked" policy to encourage their teen or young adult to call home if they are in an urgent situation and need help.

5

Sex, Tech, and Hooking Up

Given how much of young people's lives are spent online, it's no surprise that parents agonize over who and what their child will encounter in digital spaces. About 95 percent of teenagers own or have access to a smartphone and, on average, children now get their first phone at about age eleven.[38] Even before they have a phone, many children have connected devices such as tablets or watches that send and receive messages.

Young people often tell me how technology has made their romantic and sexual lives better. They talk about coming out on Instagram with huge support from friends, learning from YouTube sex educators that masturbation is nothing to feel ashamed about, and forming online friendships that offer hope in times of loneliness. Yet, most young people have also weathered painful online problems such as bullying, stalking, sexual harassment, and/or having images of them shared without permission—too often done by someone they thought they could trust.

This chapter highlights some of the most common and consequential sexuality-related issues facing young people as they navigate digital spaces, from sexting to online sexual harassment and image-based abuse to dating/ hookup apps. My approach to these sensitive topics remains grounded in core ideas woven throughout the book, such as body sovereignty, healthy relationships, care, and kindness, as well as consent. It's also set against a backdrop that honors the incredible journey young people navigate as they move through adolescence and into young adulthood, times in which they are working to establish their own identity, create strong friendships, and explore romantic and/or sexual feelings.

As parents, we are often trying to strike the right balance between supporting our kids' growing independence while keeping them safe. Online spaces can feel especially fraught. Kristina, Susan, and I have combed through our professional experiences to identify areas that parents simply must know about to have more informed conversations with their kids and figure out this balancing act.

TAKING AND SHARING SEXUAL IMAGES

When sexual text messages or nude images (whether photos or videos) are texted to one another, they're often referred to as *sexts*. Given how common sexting is—15 percent of teenagers have sent a sext and 27 percent have received one[39]—combined with how often adults panic about adolescent sexuality, it's no surprise that teens and their families land in difficult situations. As teens grow into young adults, sharing nudes becomes more prevalent. About half of young adults have sexted at least once, often involving the sharing of nude or partially nude images (not just sexy messages). Students may view the consensual sharing of these images as flirtation, a turn-on, or as a reflection of trust, intimacy, or love; however, sexting can also be pressured or coerced.

Taking, sharing, and/or forwarding nude, partially nude, or other sexual images is one of the most common digital challenges affecting young people. For simplicity, we'll refer to these as "nude images" or "nudes" even though many involve partial nudity. The biggest concern is nonconsensual sharing of such images. About 12 percent of teenagers (and 9 percent of nine- to twelve-year-olds)[40] have forwarded a nude image without permission from the person depicted. Not all nonconsensual sharing is meant to be hurtful,[41] but that doesn't change the potential harm. Sometimes people forward sexual images because they see sexting as such a normative part of life that they don't even give it a second thought. Other times people nonconsensually share images to hurt someone's reputation or publicly shame them. Mostly, students share images with their friends in order to look cool.

However, there are potential social and legal implications of creating, sending, or asking for nude pictures even when they aren't shared with others. Some people get into trouble at school and/or with the law for having asked for or shared a nude image, pressured someone to take one, and even for consensual sharing of images. It's important to make your child aware of the effects of their actions on others as well as the possible consequences.

Setting Rules Related to Sex and Technology Use

It's helpful to be open with your child about rules and expectations for technology. Ideally, families will work together to agree upon technology rules as well as whether, and to what extent, parents will monitor or check in on their kids' use of smartphones, social media, and pornography. Being transparent and collaborative about rules accomplishes two important things: (1) it helps kids to feel trusted, and (2) it grows their skills and independence. Whatever rules you come up with together, make sure they are realistic, rooted in trust, and transparent.

Studies on adolescent sexting (as well as other adolescent behaviors) show that parenting style matters. Similar to being an "askable" parent when it comes to talking about sex, having a warm and supportive relationship and being instructive about sexting (having open parent-child conversations, discussing online safety together) is more effective than taking a restrictive approach, such as forbidding technology use or imposing lots of parent-directed rules. For teenagers, a growing sense of autonomy is important to how they feel about themselves. Engaging your child in thoughtful conversations about online safety also teaches them skills they will need during adulthood.

If you plan to monitor your child's technology use, say that you will, and describe why. As your child grows older, you will likely be able to monitor their technology use less frequently, or not at all. Saying that you won't monitor their device use, but then doing it anyway, is a violation of trust. Families need to find common ground that works for everyone and aims to grow independence and trust.

SEXTING, LAWS, AND OTHER CONSEQUENCES

Laws related to sexting and nude images vary widely. While some states have sexting-specific statutes, many don't, and the sharing of nude images (even consensually between minors) may be a crime analyzed under the state's statute(s) related to child pornography (or child sexual abuse material, the term that researchers, government agencies, and advocacy organizations are increasingly adopting, as it highlights the material's abusive aspects[42]).

Yet, consensual sexting—whether sending messages or sexual images—is now recognized as both prevalent and a developmentally normative form of adolescent sexual expression. International experts have even called for the widespread decriminalization of consensual adolescent sexting of images, noting, "Just like sex, sexting should be considered a health and developmental issue, not a legal issue."[43] Instead of prosecuting teens for sexting, many prosecutors agree to place them into diversionary programs that educate teens and, upon successful completion, avoid a criminal conviction.

In some places, laws related to consensual sexting between adolescents have been relaxed (sometimes decriminalizing it or considering it a misdemeanor), whereas in other places these images may be treated as child sexual abuse material and categorized as a felony. It's important to learn about the laws where you live and talk with your child about them, especially if they have access to a phone, computer, or other device with a camera. Experts suggest that schools should provide young people with information about sexting and image sharing (especially because many schools now require students to use tablets and other connected devices during the school day and/or for homework),[44] but this rarely happens. And when photos are shared on school grounds, school leaders often must report the behavior and get involved, which can get messy.

Even when sharing images doesn't lead to school suspension, expulsion, or legal trouble (and often it does not), when sexual messages or images are passed around it can lead to teasing, harassment, blackmail, anxiety, and/or depression. Girls and young women overwhelmingly bear the brunt of these consequences, and especially bisexual women, who are more likely to report sending sexual images as well as receiving unwanted sexual images as compared to lesbians and heterosexual women.[45] In rare but tragic cases, some people have ended their own lives after their images were shared without their permission, whether to a handful of peers or widely on the internet.[46] People can be cruel. And unfortunately, once someone has shared or uploaded a nude image, there is no telling where it will end up or how many people will see it. This uncertainty contributes to the anxiety that many people experience when they learn that nude pictures of them have been nonconsensually shared with others.

I remember how nervous and vulnerable one of my students said she felt after she had allowed her ex-boyfriend to take a series of videos of them having sex. Although she acknowledged agreeing to let him take the videos, she also said she never felt good about it. "It was always his idea," she said. "He used his phone to take the videos, and he stored them on his laptop, meaning he had total control over them." Even while they were together, she said, she would wake up worrying what would happen if her boyfriend lost his phone or had his laptop stolen. When they had disagreements, she hesitated to speak her mind because she worried about upsetting him to the point where he might take things out on her by sharing their private images.

After they broke up, she worried whether he would keep his word and delete the videos.

But it's not just exes who sometimes share such images; Kristina and Susan have seen numerous instances in which a student's current partner (or close friend) was the one who passed around nude pictures without consent. Some of my students—even young men who come across as shy and sensitive and describe waiting to have sex until they find someone they truly like—have told me that they've showed their friends the nude images that others have sent to them. They don't feel good about their actions but describe feeling pressured to prove (especially if they haven't yet had sex) that there are people out there who do, in fact, desire them.

The best defense against having nude images shared without permission is not taking or sharing them in the first place, even with a trusted partner. This is not to blame the victim. If we accept that young people are the rulers of their own bodies, then we need to acknowledge that some young people may enjoy expressing their sexuality through photographs. But because non-consensual image sharing can be so harmful to young people, it's important for parents to talk with their kids about this possibility with the hope of getting them to think twice about taking and/or sharing images.

What Do I Say?

Common Questions About Sexting and Nudes

Q: How do I even start talking with my child about nude images?
Start with foundational conversations that are focused on boundaries, consent, and picture-taking. You can tell your child to:

- **Ask before taking pictures of others.** Model this by asking "Can I take a picture of you?" before snapping away. Sometimes children don't feel like being the center of attention; asking permission shows consideration. For older kids who sleep over at friends' houses, emphasize that they should not take pictures of people who are sleeping. For teens and young adults, add that they shouldn't take pictures of friends who are too drunk to consent.

- **Ask before sharing pictures of others—even nonsexual images.** All too many kids have been upset to learn that someone at school, on the bus, or at an extracurricular activity had taken pictures or video of them without permission and then posted the images to social media. Sometimes the images were accompanied by demeaning comments, making others feel made fun of and powerless. If you learn that your child has done this, explain the problem, make sure the images are removed, and ask them how they might be able to repair any harm they've caused. Remind them about the importance of being the ruler of one's own body, and that it's not fair to post pictures of others without permission, nor is it kind to make fun of them.

- **Only take pictures of people when they're dressed.** For young children, say that we don't take pictures of people when they're not dressed: no nude breasts, penises, vulvas, or butts in pictures. For older kids, give more details about how this includes no sharing (or taking) nudes—no matter who is in the picture (friend, crush, dating partner, ex). For kids who are old enough to understand, say that while it is normal to be curious about and enjoy looking at one another's body, it is often against the law to take, share, or forward images of minors. If your child has access to a connected device (their own, yours, or one of their friends), this conversation should start right away. Parents of even very young children have told me stories about their child taking and sharing pictures of their butt, penis, and/or vulva with friends, even accidentally sharing these images with cousins and grandparents. Exploring and having fun with one's body is typical childhood play, so care should be taken not to shame children; at the same time, parents need to be aware of the challenges of typical play combined with technological access. These instances are often a wake-up call for parents to monitor device use and/or have needed conversations.

Q: At what age should we talk about taking, sharing, or receiving nude images?

It's wise to start a conversation about taking and sharing pictures of bodies if your child has a phone or other device that can take or receive pictures and/or if they spend unsupervised time with friends or family who have such devices. For many families this will be between ages eight and twelve; for some, it may be as young as age five. How much to share depends on your child's age, developmental readiness, unsupervised time with device access, whether they're romantically hanging out with or dating someone, as well as the activities they're engaging in online (social media use, online video games). For younger kids, talk in terms of not taking or sharing pictures of nude or mostly nude bodies. For older kids who know about sex, you can also use the term *sexting* since they may hear it from peers. Preparing your child can help prevent problems later. If they play online video games, familiarize yourself with parental controls and safety features, consider disabling the chat function, and discuss online safety together. This includes not clicking on images or links sent by strangers.

Q. What should I tell my older kids about sexting?

As children get their own devices, are around peers with devices, and/or reach adolescence, direct conversations are needed. Here are some key messages to consider:

- **Most teenagers don't send sexts.** Although some may believe that "everybody sexts," it's not true: 85 percent of teenagers have never sent a sext and three-quarters have never received one.

- **Acknowledge that curiosity and exploration are natural while describing the very real potential consequences of sharing nude images.** These include harassment, anxiety, bullying, and legal repercussions. Youth who are aware of the potential legal consequences of exchanging images and videos are less likely to sext.[47]

- **Don't ask for nude images.** Too often, people shame the person who sent a nude image, even though most people send images because they were asked, pressured, guilted, or threatened into doing so. Let your child know that asking others for nude images puts other people in a difficult spot. Ask your child, "What if your or their phone gets lost or stolen? What if you having their image causes them to feel anxious or lose sleep?" In many places, asking a minor (even if they're a peer) to send a nude image may be against school policy or flat-out illegal.

- **Don't share, or encourage others to share, nude images.** Again, sharing nude images can be harmful to other people, perpetuates peers' feelings of being unsafe, is usually against school policies, and (if the images involve minors) is often against the law too. Also, ask them not to stand by or laugh if their friends post, forward, or show off other people's pictures. Remind them of the Golden Rule—to treat other people the way they want to be treated.

- **Adults should never ask minors for nude images.** Things can get muddy with, say, an eighteen-year-old (adult) and their seventeen-year-old (minor) dating partner. Make sure your child understands this and that you (and they) are aware of applicable laws. Specifically, tell them not to ask minors for nude images under any circumstances, even if they are close in age and the other person is someone they're dating. If they receive sexual images from a minor, they should delete them immediately.

- **If someone asks your child to share nude images with them, let them know they can use you as an excuse.** They can say, "No way. My parents have a strict rule against nudes and they monitor my device use." Even if you don't monitor, some teens find it easier to get out of sticky peer situations if they can invoke family rules and oversight.

- **Although it's wrong and unfair, the sexual double standard often applies.** Girls and young women who send nudes often experience slut-shaming, bullying, or reputational harm. Boys and young men who do so are less likely to experience negative consequences and may even score popularity points.[48] A girl's nude gets her called a slut, whereas a guy's friends may react to his nude by calling it "hilarious."[49] Encourage your child to show care for others, including classmates who may be more vulnerable to bullying, teasing, and harm, such as girls and LGBTQ+ peers. Whatever your child's gender, if they are popular among their peers, they may be able to set the tone, showing that nonconsensual sharing of nudes, slut-shaming, and bullying are neither cool nor acceptable.

- **Speak up if you learn that peers are taking or sharing nude images without permission.** Ask your child to come to you if they hear of this happening among their friends or classmates. Examples include showing nudes to friends, secretly taking nude pictures in a locker room or while hooking up, forwarding sexts without permission, or posting nude images online.

- **Ask your child to come to you if they're in a bind.** Be clear that, even if they did something you asked them not to do (such as if they took, sent, or forwarded a nude image to a peer, or sent one to an adult), you're there for them.

The key word is *educate*. Fear tactics don't usually work and may cause harm, including making your child feel that there's no way out if they've already sent a nude image to someone. This may make them feel isolated and more vulnerable to blackmail. Treat your teen as the competent, capable, almost adult that they are. Ask what they've heard about requesting or sending sexual images, share what you've learned, and calmly explain the potential emotional, social, and legal consequences. Let them know you're here to support them as they navigate this tricky terrain.

Q. What if my teenager unexpectedly receives a sexual image from someone?

As about one in four teenagers will receive a nude image, having a plan in place helps. Tell your child that, if they receive a nude image from someone, they should delete the image immediately. If they tell you that someone has sent them a nude image, thank them for coming to you. If they don't know the person (or don't know them well), they might want to block the person on their phone. If the sender is a staff member or teacher at your child's school, contact the school and local law enforcement (who you can also contact if the sender is an adult outside the school). Ask your child to let you know if it happens again and that you'll help them figure it out.

Q. What if my child is being asked for nude images?

Offer to develop a plan with your child to combat pressure to send nudes and check in about it every now and then. Some kids choose to block someone who asks them for nudes. Others take a different tactic, especially if the person asking for nudes is a friend or dating partner. Some teens, when asked for "dirty pictures," have replied with pictures of muddy boots; when asked for pictures of breasts, have sent pictures of chicken breasts; or when asked for a "dick pic" have texted back a Richard Nixon meme. They make a joke of it and do not send nude images of themselves or others. If your child's school has a policy against students asking for nudes or sexts, they can screenshot the request and show it to school leadership to nip things in the bud. Emphasize that asking someone for nudes after they have said no, or trying to guilt or pressure someone into sending nudes, is a huge red flag in a friendship or relationship. They might want to reconsider whether they want to be spending time with that person. Finally, if the person asking for nudes is an adult, tell your child that you need to know right away—especially if that person is trying to get them to move their online conversation to a different platform or app, or if they have asked to meet your child offline. Contact the authorities to report adults who are asking for nude images of your child.

Q. How can I support my teen if a sexual image of them has been shared without permission?

If someone has nonconsensually shared your child's sexual image, thank your kid for letting you know. Reassure them that you love them, that you're there to support them, and that you can get through this together. Listen to and validate their feelings by reflecting back what they've shared with you ("You're feeling betrayed") rather than brushing their feelings away with an "Everything will be fine."

See if you can get more information: Who has seen or has a copy of the image? Take a cue from your kid about what they want to do. Some parents address this with one another, parent to parent. Others contact counsel to determine legal options, including how to find out where else the image may have been shared. While you don't want to minimize the potential harm, try to focus on your teen as a whole human being—someone with hobbies, dreams, interests, school, and other things that deserve attention. Obsessing over the image may make things worse, so remember to ask about other aspects of your child's life too. Finally, help them come up with a plan for how to respond if someone brings up the nude: they might prefer to ignore comments or else they might have a response ready to go such as, "The real problem is that Person X shared that picture without my permission. That was wrong."

Q. What do I do if I learn my teen has been sexting with another teen?
Even though most teens don't sext or send nude images to their peers, many do, so it's wise to be prepared for the possibility. Try to:

- **Find your calm.** As Dr. Jeff Temple, a professor and psychologist at the University of Texas Medical Branch, put it: "It's a fairly normative behavior; it doesn't mean your kid is deviant or in a life of crime . . . it means they're interested in their sexuality and sex."[50] Exploring romantic and sexual feelings is a normal part of adolescent development.
- **Express curiosity.** Instead of "What were you thinking?" consider "I understand that many people sext and for lots of different reasons. I'm curious how this came about." Some people sext because they want to, others because they feel pressured, coerced, or worry their crush might lose interest if they don't. Some crave positive feedback to boost their self-esteem. Learning about the context will help you better understand your child.
- **Avoid shaming them.** They're probably mortified that you've stumbled across their sexts. Talking with young people about the potential consequences of their behavior can be balanced with respect for them as sexual beings.
- **Ask your child to delete any nude pictures they have of themselves or other minors.** They should ask the other teen to delete any

images of them too. Laws vary, but it's better to be safe than sorry when it comes to nude images of minors—hit delete.

- **Tell your child to stop asking for, sending, or accepting nude pictures.** If they resist or say that they and their friend or partner are going to continue to sext even though it's illegal where you live, you may need to take away your kid's devices for a while and/or engage the other teenager's parent(s) to come up with a plan. If their behavior was legal but not in keeping with your family's technology agreement, consider occasional spot checks to make sure no nude pictures are being exchanged.. Kristina and Susan have had cases where law enforcement, prosecutors, and judges wanted to know why parents did not deny access to devices or utilize home internet filters once they knew that their child was accessing images of minors even when the minor was a friend or partner.

- **Know when to seek help.** If police contact your child for questioning, contact counsel immediately.

IMAGE-BASED SEXUAL ABUSE

Image-based sexual abuse (IBSA) is an umbrella term that includes aggressive, abusive, or coercive acts that involve images such as pictures and video, and applies to both digital images and physical copies of images. IBSA is on the spectrum of sexual violence; its intent is to harm. Images are used to stalk, embarrass, threaten, harass, slut-shame, or blackmail the person depicted in the images (often called *sextortion*, which about 5 percent of teenagers have experienced). Without permission—and often without the subject's knowledge—these images may be shared with friends, partners, exes, or on the internet, or posted around school. IBSA is sometimes called *revenge porn*, though many believe that the term should be retired as it centers the motives of the abuser and suggests something consensual occurred by using the word *porn*.[51] The term *image-based sexual abuse* more clearly highlights that this is an act of harm or abuse.

Kristina and Susan have seen many cases of IBSA where an ex-partner threatens to disseminate nude pictures to an employer, family members, or on the internet, sometimes to extort their former partner for money and other times just to punish their partner for ending the relationship. Because IBSA is so widespread, there are many professionals, including within law firms, whose work involves removing content from the internet. Unfortunately, once a person shares nude images, control over those images is lost. Regaining control can be a costly, exhausting, and sometimes unproductive venture.

IBSA has detrimental effects on victims. Sometimes people who share or post images without permission minimize their behavior, saying it was "just a joke." While many teenagers may not understand the potential legal implications of their behavior, most people realize that sharing images without permission is not kind and would be upsetting to those pictured. Passing photos or videos around is not a small thing; it shouldn't be downplayed or excused as a joke. Be clear with your teen that nonconsensually sharing, posting, or threatening to share others' nude images is not acceptable.

THE PAINFUL REALITIES OF TAKING AND SHARING NUDE PICTURES

As a sixteen-year-old who had never before been in trouble at school, Lucas was shocked to find himself facing expulsion, and so were his parents. Yet, after forwarding nude pictures of his classmate Sophia to his friends, an expulsion hearing and criminal investigation are precisely where Lucas found himself. When a teacher overheard Lucas and some of his classmates talking about the photos, Lucas was sent to the principal's office. Lucas confessed to everything—to both the principal and the local police officers who were called to the school to seize Lucas's phone. Not only did Lucas have nude pictures of Sophia on his phone, he also had nude pictures of other girls from school. The next day, flanked by lawyers, Lucas learned that although the nude pictures depicted girls who were his own age, the photos technically constituted child sexual abuse materials, since the girls in the pictures were all under eighteen. And by sharing the photos with other boys in his school, Lucas had technically disseminated what was considered "child pornography,"* according to the laws where he lived.

Lucas's parents were shocked that the principal would question their son without calling them first. However, school officials are generally not legally obligated to wait for parents to arrive at school before questioning a student. His parents were also in shock that Lucas had shared the images in the first place. One can only imagine the stress, anxiety, and embarrassment he caused Sophia and the other girls who learned that their nude images had been passed around by people they had trusted.

Every year, many teens (and even some older elementary-aged children) find themselves facing juvenile charges and other consequences, including suspension or expulsion from schools, for sharing nude images. In smaller towns, the families are often friends, making the situation even messier. At private schools, students are sometimes encouraged to withdraw from school rather than risk being expelled. Too often, the victims—who are usually girls or young women—are harassed online or at school. They may be slut-shamed by their peers or notice classmates giving them sexualized "head to toe" looks as they pass in the hallway, often to intimidate or bully them. Some don't feel like they can ever return to their school. Others do, but their mental health spirals from being victimized (first from the non-consensual sharing and then by their peers), leading to additional problems such as cutting themselves, eating disorders, or substance abuse. Even when young people feel supported by their friends and classmates, they may wonder how far their picture traveled: *Is it posted online somewhere? Do other kids in their community have a copy?* If your child's images have been nonconsensually shared, first and foremost they need love and support—not shame or

---

* As noted earlier, we acknowledge that the term "child pornography" is no longer used by many governmental and advocacy organizations, but it does remain the legal term in many places and is thus the term we use here.

blame. Adolescent sexual exploration is normal. Trusting a good friend or partner is nothing to be embarrassed about; if your child's trust was misplaced, that's not their fault, even if it is a painful lesson to learn.

Cases involving nude images aren't always about sex. Hayden was an eighth grader who found himself in trouble following a class trip to Chicago. One night in the hotel room, Hayden and his friends had decided to compare their penis sizes. While it's common for kids to compare their bodies, especially around puberty, Hayden and his friends didn't just compare their penises; they took pictures to see who had the largest penis. The boys even took a photo of the penis of a classmate who was sleeping at the time. School officials later found out what the boys had done, confiscated their phones, and initiated the expulsion process. Here, once again, there was a parallel criminal investigation for child sexual abuse materials (which Hayden described as "dick pics," even at his young age) and the eighth graders' decision to (nonconsensually) take a photo of the genitals of the boy who was sleeping.

Taking a proactive approach to these conversations is important: Make sure to talk with your child about never taking nude images of other kids (especially without consent). Also, review your family's rules and remind them of ways to resist peer pressure and focus on kindness before your child attends a sleepover or overnight class trip or sporting trip, where group dynamics may become challenging.

ONLINE VOYEURISM

One form of IBSA involves people (mostly men) nonconsensually sharing images (usually of women) on email lists or websites. The pictures may be ones that they took with or without permission, or they may be pictures that the victim once sent to them and the recipient then nonconsensually uploaded to the site or sent on the listserv. Some listservs or sites are specific to certain high schools, colleges, sports teams, fraternities, or the military. Others are organized among friends. Often, group members can comment on the pictures, such as rating them in terms of how hot or "slutty" they appear.

While technically these sites are called *online image-based evaluative voyeurism (OIBEV)*, people usually refer to them as *slutpages*, reflecting the misogyny underlying these sites. In one study, about half of male college athletes and 60 percent of fraternity men surveyed reported that they'd visited a slutpage to view and/or post nude images of classmates.[52] These sites are popular and participating in them can sometimes feel like a form of belonging or bonding (but at the expense of the women whose pictures have been posted).

If you haven't yet talked with your teen or young adult child about these sites, now is the time. Ask them what they may have heard about slutpages. Ask them not to visit such pages. Also, discuss how visiting or adding to these sites relates to their values, their views on women, their integrity, and the person they want to become—not to mention the potential harm to victims (including anxiety, depression, concerns for one's personal safety, and even thoughts of suicide). There are also serious legal implications of creating, maintaining, or adding images to a shared site like these. In a well-known college campus case, a fraternity member had concerns about images that had been shared online, in a closed Facebook group maintained by members of his fraternity.[53] It was clear to this young man that the pictures he'd seen online had likely been shared without the women's consent and that doing so was wrong. Presumably following his conscience, he printed out the pages and brought them to the police. Criminal and campus investigations followed, as well as demonstrations on campus, with students understandably expressing their anger at their classmates' behavior and demanding accountability.

STANDING UP AGAINST MISOGYNY

Most women have been catcalled or had strangers say something sexual to them. About half of women have been demeaned by someone calling them a bitch, slut, or whore.[54] Even among middle school girls, 43 percent have experienced sexual harassment, with one in five having been sexually touched, grabbed, or pinched in an unwanted way.[55] In *The Emotional Lives of Teenagers*, psychologist Dr. Lisa Damour describes how sexual harassment often picks up in the middle school years as many boys notice that: (1) their masculinity may be judged by their size, strength, speed, and accomplishments and (2) girls—who tend to be developmentally more mature—are often taller, stronger, faster, and further ahead intellectually as compared to boys at these ages. Middle school is a time when young people are going through puberty and overcome with hormones. Boys of all sexual orientations often feel like they need to be seen as traditionally masculine. Those who are feeling insecure about being upstaged by girls may attempt to manage their distress by trying to shift the power balance in harmful ways, such as making derogatory comments about girls' bodies or sexuality or even grabbing their breasts or butts. This does not excuse this sexual harassment, but understanding this potential pathway can give parents and schools insights into prevention.

Despite long-standing problems with sexual harassment and misogyny, most adults do very little to prevent, address, or stand up to it among young people. About three-quarters of youth say that they've never had a conversation with their parents about how not to sexually harass others.[56] The absence of official reports about school-based sexual harassment suggests that many incidents may be swept under the rug ("that's just his way of showing he likes you").[57] Yet, we all benefit when we work to prevent misogyny and sexual harassment and then stand up to it when it occurs, creating conditions for a kinder, more equitable world. Here are some steps you can take to help your child (of any gender) do so:

- **Help them learn to tolerate distress.** Learning to manage difficult feelings—such as envy, insecurity, fear, and anger—is a key life skill. When you sense your child may be feeling powerless, angry, or emasculated, help them name and tolerate those feelings so they're less likely to push them away in harmful ways. Naming and validating their feelings can help ("It seems like you're feeling hurt") as can sharing the benefits of taking slow breaths to calm one's body, using positive self-talk, and asking for hugs or one-on-one time together to foster connection and feel supported.

- **Talk about power dynamics.** Be aware of times that your child tries to make other people feel small so they can feel big. Adults sometimes do this, too, by being condescending or gossiping about someone's appearance or behavior. Becoming aware of power dynamics within our own families and friend groups is the first step toward being thoughtful about how power is used.

- **Name misogyny and sexual harassment.** Share that people of all genders harass others and that even comments meant as jokes can be hurtful and harassing. Most young women say that catcalling makes them feel scared, offended, angry, or powerless; it doesn't feel like a compliment.[58] Even so-called locker room talk, like joking about penis size or describing sexual encounters with a classmate, can make people feel uncomfortable.

- **Emphasize that sending unsolicited nudes is not okay.** Most young adult women who have used dating/hookup apps say that another user has sent them a sexually explicit image or message that they didn't ask for.[59] Young gay and bisexual men also describe commonly receiving unsolicited dick pics or nudes. While some people enjoy seeing nude images, others are turned off or feel threatened, which makes communication and consent critical. Always ask before sending (and again: when nude images are sent at all, it should be between adults—not minors).

Because sexual harassment and misogyny are large societal issues, tackling them shouldn't just be on your shoulders. Ask your child's school what they do to address these topics, such as through faculty and staff professional development. Also, how are sexual harassment and misogyny addressed in middle school or high school curricula, such as in courses related to ethics, media, communication, or health education?

Finally, be observant. Look for teachable moments, like if your child use phrases like "bros over hos," spends time on pickup-artist sites, says someone throws like a girl or acts like a pussy, or posts pictures from a party whose theme was "office hos and CEOs." If you overhear your child or their friends call someone a "whore," ask what that means to them. Calling someone a slut or whore is a way of dehumanizing someone, which may make it easier for someone to feel entitled to pressure, coerce, or force them into having sex. Thinking of someone as a slut or whore also makes it all too easy to assume they're lying if they say they've been sexually assaulted. So, stop that language in its tracks—even if they say, "It's just a joke." Engage your child in thoughtful dialogue by asking why they and their friends joke or bond in those ways, or how sexist comments are similar to or different from racist comments. Encourage your child to think about the effects of their comments on others and to find power in the idea that they can help end misogyny rather than perpetuate it.

DEEPFAKES

Even if you're not familiar with the term *deepfake*, you've probably seen some version of one. Deepfakes are realistic-looking videos made using artificial intelligence. Sometimes deepfake videos are lighthearted, such as viral deepfakes that superimpose actor Nicolas Cage's face on the bodies of other famous actors and actresses. There are also serious concerns that deepfake videos of political leaders could be used to spread disinformation or provoke wars. However, the vast majority of deepfake videos—about 96 percent—appear to be pornographic in nature.[60] People use pictures or videos of people (often celebrities, exes, or women who rejected them), combined with artificial intelligence, to create real-looking sexual images. That is, they superimpose images of people's faces onto the bodies of pornographic actors, usually without permission.

Nonconsensual deepfake pornography is a form of IBSA, and women are overwhelmingly the victims. Highly sophisticated technical skills aren't even needed; online tools and forums make it easy to create deepfakes either by oneself or with the help of an online stranger.[61] Laws are constantly having to catch up to new technologies, and as of this writing, people who have been victimized by deepfake IBSA do not always have legal recourse. Around the world, there are efforts to change this so that people can be held accountable for creating deepfakes. If someone in your family is victimized in this way, contact legal counsel to see what help may be available.

SOCIAL MEDIA

Social media sites and apps are like celebrities; those that are popular today may be old news by next year. While most young people used to hang out on Facebook, they later fled to Twitter, Instagram, and Snapchat, then migrated to TikTok, WhatsApp, and BeReal. It's anyone's guess where young people will flock to next. Instead of focusing on specific sites, it can be helpful for parents to think about providing their child with more general guidance. That way, no matter which app is in or out, they can learn to approach social media in a healthier way.

Although it can be easy to swim in our own fears about young people and social media, there are upsides. These include feeling more connected to friends and family, becoming politically engaged, practicing social skills, finding community, and happiness boosts from looking at cute pictures of kittens. Young people who find it difficult to articulate their feelings in person may find it easier to open up online, where they can take time to describe their thoughts.

Social media also fills huge gaps in school-based sex education. Many of my college students credit YouTube and TikTok sex educators with helping them learn the basics back when they were in high school. And for some young people, social media sites provide the first opportunity to see someone who looks like them talking about sex. It can be powerful for young

Black women to learn from Black sex educators. Similarly, it's affirming for young disabled people (or those dating someone with a disability) to learn firsthand from disabled sex educators.

Unfortunately, social media also presents challenges. When people spend gobs of time on social media, they're more likely to feel depressed and/or anxious, get less sleep, have poorer body image, and exercise too little.[62] Teenage girls are especially hit hard by social media's effects on mental health and body image. This can leave them feeling vulnerable to pressure to share nude pictures in exchange for affirmation or affection.

To mitigate these effects, parents can:

- **Encourage kids to delay getting on social media and, once on, limit their time using such sites.** As a parent, set an example by stepping away from screens when possible. Also, many devices have settings that allow people to set limits on how long they spend on certain apps or sites. Some parents take the Wait Until 8th pledge (WaitUntil8th.org), committing to delay giving their child a smartphone until eighth grade or later (basic phones still offer the ability to call and text so they can be in touch).

- **Help your child reflect on how social media impacts them.** How do they feel after spending time on certain social media platforms? Are there particular people or celebrity accounts they follow that leave them feeling unattractive, poor, or unpopular? Have they considered unfollowing those accounts or not checking the app as often? In comparison, how do they feel after going to dance class, playing sports, or spending time with family or friends? Where do they feel happiest and like they can be themselves? Many people try taking a break from certain apps to see how it changes the way they feel.

- **Urge your child to keep their photos private and to be mindful about what they share online.** Several of my students have described how anonymous strangers have copied images that my students posted to social media sites (often images of them in swimsuits) and then used those images to impersonate them on OnlyFans or a similar subscription site; even worse, the stranger then messaged their friends and family, urging them to check out their OnlyFans site.

- **Describe how you make your own choices.** This can be as simple as casually saying, "I realized that by following _____ (fill in the blank with a certain celebrity or influencer), I started comparing myself to them, which made me feel bad. Now that I've unfollowed them, I feel calmer and more comfortable with myself and my body."

- **Ask your child to let you know immediately if someone asks them for sexy or nude pictures.** The requested pictures may be of them in their bra, underwear, swimsuit, or nude, or could be of them doing something sexual. I've heard from parents whose teens have been approached online by adults, sometimes offering hundreds of dollars in exchange for nude images. For some, this has occurred via social media direct messages (which are private) or online gaming platforms. According to the National Center for Missing and Exploited Children, online exploitation attempts (which includes attempts to get kids to take or send nude images, meet face-to-face, or engage in sexual conversations) are rising, and nearly doubled from 2019 to 2020.[63] These pictures may be used to blackmail kids into sending more pictures, or even into meeting up offline, which makes them vulnerable to sexual assault or being trafficked for sex (something that has also dramatically increased in recent years).

- **Ask your child to let you know if an adult adds them as a friend or begins to "like" their posts.** Even if the age difference doesn't seem large, there are concerns about adults and minors friending one another on social media. I've heard from parents about too many blurred lines and unsafe situations that have happened between young people and their adult camp counselors, coaches, or community mentors. Parents should ask their child to let them know if or when an adult friends or follows them, begins liking their posts, texts them, or direct messages them.

- **Remind your child that potential colleges/universities and employers look at social media.** Ask your child to apply the following filters when posting online: Is this an image that I am proud of others viewing? Does this statement accurately depict me as an individual? Also remind them that fake or secondary accounts (which many teens have in order to post photos out of their parents' sight) may not be as private as they think.

- **Talk about privacy in relation to online safety.** Common Sense Media offers parent/teen guides about social media and location-based services, including guidance for how to adjust these settings in various social media apps and sites. Showing one's location can put kids at risk for in-person stalking, harassment, assault, or sex trafficking, especially if they've been posting images to acquaintances, to social media, or the wider world. Also make sure that young people understand how easy it is for others to figure out who they are and where they live, often with very little effort, even when location is turned off (e.g., by noticing details in pictures such as a school T-shirt or that most of their comments come from teenagers who go to the same school).

Because social media is here to stay, it's important to help your child learn to live with it. The good news is, young people are eager for guidance from adults they trust. Trey, a nineteen-year-old agender student, shared with me that, although their own parents weren't particularly communicative, their best friend's parents were open, knowledgeable, and always made them feel accepted. Trey said that one time, when they were about eight or nine years old, their friend's parents sat them and their friend down, "explaining to us in terms that we could understand that there are scary and dangerous things out there, so don't take the risk. [Their friend's parents] said, 'You know, don't be clicking on links from people. Don't be giving people your information.' Um, you know, giving us that knowledge about the internet to be safe." At the time, the parents were cautioning them about connecting with adults while playing *Minecraft*. However, the overarching message would support Trey for years to come.

VIDEO CHATTING WITH STRANGERS

Perhaps you've heard of video chat sites like Omegle and Chatroulette (though there are others), which people use to connect, randomly, with strangers on the internet. While sometimes described as a way to meet interesting people online, many of my women students share that they've mostly seen adult men exposing their genitals and/or masturbating on such video chat sites. What's more, these women describe having used these sites not recently as adults but at much younger ages (as older elementary or middle school students), while at sleepover parties or hanging out at friends' homes.

Trey remembers these sites, too, but fortunately the warnings they took to heart from their best friend's parents served them well, even years later when their friends were videochatting with strangers online at sleepovers. While they recall some of their childhood friends being upset to see adult men expose themselves online, Trey heeded the warning and chose not to watch. It's not just Trey or my students, however, who have had these experiences; in 2022, *Mother Jones* published an article describing other young girls' experiences seeing adult men expose themselves online, also on video chat sites. Even worse, the *Mother Jones* article described rare but horrible situations where adult men moved the chats to other platforms and then convinced young people to send nude pictures or even to meet offline, leading to sexual assault.

The bad news is that too many young people encounter adults online in sexual contexts. The good news is that young people want guidance from their parents (and even trusted friends' parents). Your support and messages of caution can go a long way. If your child uses social media, talk about these issues with them. Ask about their familiarity with video chat sites. Also, reach out to other parents to start a conversation; when parents can make each other aware of what kids sometimes see online, they may decide how they can band together to limit unsupervised device use when friends are hanging out, level up their use of content filters, and/or guide their kids to safer and more fun uses of social media.

SUBSCRIPTION CONTENT PLATFORMS

The COVID-19 pandemic brought about a rise in the visibility of subscription-based content platforms (one of the most well-known being OnlyFans) through which people can sell and/or purchase content, some of which is sexual. Content creators who offer sexual images may do so because they enjoy sexually expressing themselves in this way, it has greater flexibility than other kinds of work, and/or because it feels safer to them than in-person sex work. Some young adults, noting that they have long shared nude images with people they were hooking up with or dating, describe feeling like it was about time they charged for their images, rather than giving them away for free.

Technically subscriptions sites are supposed to be for adults; however, there have been reports of minors finding ways to access subscription sites to view and/or sell content (sometimes by using an adult relative's identification). Also, young people need to know that these sites are not as private as they may feel. People sometimes nonconsensually copy and share images (without permission), which can lead to IBSA. Also, users on subscription sites sometimes try to exploit content creators. Young people tell stories of being asked to show more and more of their bodies, perform more explicit sex acts, and/or meet offline for sex. And some young people may find it difficult to resist the offer of hundreds or thousands of dollars for more risqué images.

Just letting your child know that you are aware of these sites can be an opportunity for discussion about what they have heard about them and how you each feel about them. Remind them, too, that people are not always who they say they are, that meeting strangers offline is risky, and that in many places exchanging sex for money may be illegal (whether they are the ones buying or paying). If you're concerned about your kid potentially accessing sites like these, it's wise to have an open conversation as well as check your family's filters or content settings.

THE RUMOR MILL

Perhaps you remember how, when you were growing up, reputations were lost in games of telephone tag and hallway whispers. By the time Monday rolled around, everyone had heard what happened at a Friday night party. These days, as connected as everyone is through texting and social media, reputations can be lost in seconds. This isn't just about girls being shamed for being flirtatious or sexually active, although that persists too. Rather, Kristina and Susan have worked on cases where students faced online accusations of sexual assault without any evidence to back up the claim. Some students have even created digital lists where they shared the names of other students who they believed had assaulted others and who they felt should be avoided at all costs. You may have heard of similar lists posted by adults, such as the Shitty Media Men list, a crowdsourced online spreadsheet that made headlines in 2017, in the midst of #MeToo.

In the student-created lists, once someone's name is posted, they may be "canceled," meaning excluded from friend groups, party invites, or Greek organizations. Their name and the allegations may get spray-painted around campus ("X is a rapist"). People have even decided to dox students, publicly posting their full names, addresses, and phone numbers online. In some instances that Kristina and Susan have seen, the named students have received threatening texts and voicemails warning them to watch their backs. Faced with threats of violence, the simple acts of walking to class or doing laundry can cause immense anxiety. It's even led to the students' parents receiving threats and feeling unsafe.

It's understandable why people may want to make such lists or share allegations they believe to be true. They may feel angry over something that happened to themselves, a friend, or an acquaintance. They may be acting out of a desire to protect others. After all, the legal system often fails victims of sexual assault—focusing on what the victim was wearing or the fact that they went up to someone's room rather than addressing the accused person's behavior. Too many people do horrible things, seemingly without consequence. That said, it's not okay to ruin reputations over unfounded rumors. Often the spray-painting and online postings are done by those who don't have firsthand knowledge of the accusations, but rather are just piling on and joining a group. In some instances, students admit to spreading rumors they didn't know much about and say that—in looking back—they should have been more thoughtful before making or sharing posts that accused people of something as serious as assault or rape.

Parents can model and encourage ethical behavior while at the same time supporting their child's concerns about justice. There can be serious consequences for hurting other people's reputations and their prospects for college, graduate school, and/or employment. Just as it's not okay to non-consensually post people's nude images online, it's also not okay to post online, without evidence, that someone is a rapist. It's important to let actual restorative justice processes, campus investigations, or legal processes play out. If your child does not feel the system is working and wants to take action, encourage them to try and effect change in a healthy, productive manner. Some students have successfully advocated for their campus to offer restorative justice programs, which feel more accessible to them than formal sexual misconduct proceedings. Others have lobbied their university to revise their sexual misconduct policies to recognize contemporary forms of sexual misconduct such as stealthing. And women legal scholars have been at the forefront of establishing laws against image-based sexual abuse.

SEXUAL HARASSMENT

Social media has made it easy to lash out at others. Young women especially have been subjected to cruel statements (and even threats of rape and murder) through social media and dating apps after declining to meet up with someone for sex, calling someone out on a crude or aggressive message, or even just not replying to messages. The Instagram account @ByeFelipe (among others) has cataloged many examples of these exchanges; check it out for a dose of reality. Many of my women college students have described abusive exchanges as the reason they quickly removed themselves from dating apps. According to the Pew Research Center, 44 percent of young adult women have had another user call them an offensive name, and 19 percent say that someone has threatened to physically harm them.[64] Kristina and Susan have seen some college campus cases involving undergraduate and graduate/professional students where women have been harassed and called names like "dumb bitch," underscoring how such harassment goes beyond dating contexts and into campus life. Some people react to rejection of any kind, whether from potential dating partners or potential employers, with threats, outrage, or plans for revenge. If you see this pattern in your child, please bring it up with a mental health professional who can support them in learning to regulate their emotions and becoming more resilient, even in the face of rejection.

Responding to Rejection

Once parents learn that their child and/or their peers are starting to date, hook up, or "catch feelings," it's wise to ask questions about what they think happens (or should happen) when someone doesn't feel that same way. Art and literature are full of stories of unrequited love, so you can borrow teachable moments from there, as well as accounts like @ByeFelipe. You might ask:

- What happens if someone says they're into a person, but that person doesn't share their feelings?
- What stories have you heard where someone has said they're not into someone or said no to dating them? What generally happens?
- How would you feel if someone ghosted you (ended all communication without explanation) after talking to you for a while or texting

you every day? What are some healthy and unhealthy ways people might put some space between them and a person they had been hanging out with?

- How would you feel if you no longer wanted to be texted and someone wouldn't listen to you?

Share that we all get rejected sometimes (especially as teenagers and young adults) and it's okay to hurt and healthy to cry. However, be clear that it's not okay to demean others or to make another person feel unsafe. Also, it is never okay to suggest someone should be raped or deserves to be raped (something some young people—especially young men—sometimes do via text or social media in response to having been rejected). As a parent, you can:

- **Encourage your child to respect others' boundaries.** If someone does not want to talk to them (or does not reply to messages, texts, or calls), they should stop reaching out and give them space.
- **Ask your child to take the high road.** Breaking up and being ghosted are painful, but that doesn't make it okay to lash out at the other person, whether online or offline.
- **Be there for them.** If you suspect your child is hurting, show up with love however you can: a call or text to say you love them, making their favorite dinner, tickets to a sports event, an extra-long hug, or one-on-one time together. Small gestures mean a lot.

ONLINE STALKING

Stalking is common, affecting about one in six women and one in seventeen men in their lifetimes, with nearly half of victims first experiencing stalking before they turn twenty-five.[65] Although people often think of stalking as happening in person, such as an ex showing up at a person's home or work, it also occurs online, and it's still scary when it occurs digitally. Online stalking can include incessantly texting someone, posting comments and messages across their social media platforms, and otherwise continuing to make contact even after being ignored or asked to stop. Nearly two-thirds of young adult women who use dating apps have had people continue to message them even after they said they weren't interested in them;[66] a message or two to try again may not seem harmful to most, but the more frequently that people make unwanted contact, the more concerning things get.

One troubling case that Kristina and Susan saw involved a toxic relationship between Cami and Zane. They dated for a while, and when Cami wanted to end the relationship, Zane had difficulty accepting the boundary. Zane texted Cami endlessly, hoping to get a response. When she did not respond, he messaged her on other platforms, emailed her multiple times, and called her repeatedly until she finally relented and communicated with him. This behavior persisted for months until Cami sought a no-contact order from her school.

While this case fit the stereotype of a man stalking a woman (and indeed that is the more common situation), stalking can occur between people of any gender or sexual orientation. Ask your child to come to you if someone is not taking no for an answer and if they need help figuring out what to do. Also encourage them to come to you if they're feeling heartbroken or rejected so that they can get the emotional support they need. Whenever your kid has had a breakup (no matter which side of it they're on), check in with them. Even if they say they're "fine" or have gotten over it, remind them of healthy ways to care for oneself after a relationship has ended.

Some helpful hints in the event your child feels concerned after a breakup or is being stalked:

- **Change passwords.** After a breakup, it's wise to change passwords for one's device(s) and to social media accounts, especially if there's any concern about stalking.

- **Step back from social media.** Any time someone is worried for their safety, it can be wise to go silent on social media or at least not post about where they're planning to be; this includes not "liking" event pages.
- **Keep everything.** If your child is being stalked, they should preserve the evidence; even if they would rather not see the person's name on their phone, they should hold on to the texts, emails, and direct messages rather than delete them. If the person stalking them posts something condescending or scary publicly (such as a comment on something they post) and they want to delete it, they should screenshot the post prior to deletion.
- **Explore options for protection.** Online stalking is often covered by campus policies, and schools may offer no-contact orders. Some even provide free legal aid to acquire a protective order that extends past campus and into the community.

DATING/HOOKUP APPS

"Don't talk to strangers" is an essential lesson that many parents teach their young children. Ironically, the children we tell not to talk to strangers often grow up to use hookup apps like Tinder, Grindr, or Bumble to meet people they don't know for dating or sex.

Although very few teenagers use dating or hookup sites to meet partners (given that technically they are for adults), about one-third of young adults have used these apps or sites. Going from meeting potential partners at school (where there's some familiarity among peers) to joining dating apps and potentially meeting complete strangers is a massive shift for young people, with both upsides and downsides. Many young adults are also living away from home for the first time, figuring out how to make good choices about who they invite into their dorm or apartment. Although opening up one's world can feel exciting, meeting strangers online sometimes results in sex that is pressured, coerced, rougher than expected, or even violent. Young women as well as gay and bisexual men are especially vulnerable to these situations. Stereotypes that men are supposed to always want and be ready for sex makes it difficult for some to feel like they can say no. Further, the desire to be seen as masculine can make it difficult for some young gay and bi men to stop sex that feels too rough, aggressive, or painful.

For apps, safety often begins with not giving out personal details (address, phone number) and with (eventually) meeting up in public first. But there are no foolproof ways of preventing sexual assault. After all, the best sexual assault prevention method is for a person to only engage in sex for which there is clear consent and to not hook up with someone who seems drunk or incapacitated. When deciding whether or not to use dating/hookup apps, it can be helpful for young people to ask themselves questions like:

- What kind of relationship am I looking for? Casual hookups? Dating? Long term?
- How can I communicate this to other people? (It's not helpful to say you're into something casual if you're truly wanting to date, or vice versa.)
- Are you in a good place, mentally, to deal with apps? If not, how else can you meet potential partners? Perhaps through friends, school, or parties?

Although meeting people through apps isn't for everyone, many young people enjoy meeting potential hookups and dating partners this way—especially if they're not into going to parties or bars. And I've been impressed at how students who learn they've tested positive for an STI will review their history on the app in order to notify recent partners that they may have been exposed and should get tested. Also, apps do have their success stories—many of us have friends or family who first met their partners or spouses online. If your young adult chooses to use apps for dating or hookups, encourage them to approach them with safety in mind—as well as prioritizing mutual consent and open communication.

Collective Wisdom

As a college professor, I tend to hear from young adults who have generally had reasonably okay (or even good, pleasurable, and exciting) experiences with consensual sexting and nudes, with some exceptions. However, Kristina and Susan regularly meet with young people who have experienced life-changing repercussions related to nonconsensual sharing of nude images. Not surprisingly, because our professional experiences differ, so do some of our perspectives on sexting and image sharing. However, we agree that parents should:

1. **Talk about technology, early and often.** From an early age, make sure your child knows to ask people before taking or sharing pictures of them and to only take pictures of people when their clothes are on.

2. **Model good digital citizenship by asking your kid before sharing pictures of them with others.** Yes, even before sending pictures to the grandparents. While this may sound extreme, it's easily done, shows respect, builds trust, and sets an example.

3. **Set ground rules.** Teenagers need independence yet still thrive on having some structure and rules in place. Decide together on reasonable rules around technology as well as what your child can expect in terms of parental monitoring or device spot checks, if you plan to do these. To learn about the pros and cons of filters as well as monitoring apps and services (such as Bark), Common Sense Media is a helpful resource.

4. **Teach healthy boundaries.** It's easier for families to navigate evolving sex/technology challenges when they ask themselves questions like: Is this an acceptable thing to do to someone I care about? Is this a red flag in my friendship or relationship? How can I clearly assert my boundaries and respect others' boundaries?

5. **Show you're there for them.** Many young people will find themselves in sticky situations when it comes to sex and technology. Often, kids are learning to use devices and the internet at the same time that their hormones are shifting and they're exploring crushes, sexuality, and love. Mistakes are likely to be made. While rules and good guidance are important, so are love and support. Be clear that, if or when problems arise, you'll be there for them.

6

Pornography and Other Sexually Explicit Media

When I started out as a sexuality educator, parents of tweens and teens mostly asked questions about how to talk with their children about puberty, delaying or becoming sexually active, birth control, condoms, and STI/HIV. Young people asked similar questions, alongside those about masturbation, sexual orientation, oral sex, and orgasm. These days, parents ask about pornography more than any other topic. This makes sense, given how young people have much more access to pornography than ever before. About 95 percent of teenagers are now online, where sexual images are widely available. A 2022 national survey of 1,358 teenagers ages thirteen to seventeen led by Common Sense Media found that three-quarters of teens had seen pornography and more than half had seen pornography by the time they were just thirteen years old. Teenagers of all genders report having first seen pornography, on average, at around eleven or twelve years old.

We shouldn't be surprised by these statistics, knowing that Pornhub is up there with Amazon and Google as one of the most visited websites. Access to pornography is easy and ubiquitous, even though child and adolescent development experts agree that exposure to pornography should be delayed for as long as possible. Kids' first exposure to pornography is usually unintentional; they may click on a link that a friend sent as a joke or stumble upon pornography while searching for information about puberty, looking up an unfamiliar term (*virgin*, *MILF*, *dildo*), or mistyping a web address. It is often said that it's easier for children to find pornography than to avoid it.

Before we dive in, I want to acknowledge the range of feelings and perspectives that we, as parents, bring to conversations about pornography and other sexually explicit media. Some people were raised to believe that viewing pornography is a common form of sexual exploration—materials meant for adults but that many young people come across without harm. Many adults recall seeing their first *Playboy* or other magazine hidden under a family member's bed. Others were raised to view pornography as something that only "perverted" people seek out. Some adults received mixed messages from friends, family, and media. If you have had positive experiences watching pornography or other sexually explicit media, you may understand why some teenagers are curious about it. For some, pornography and other sexually explicit media have contributed to their understanding of themselves as sexual beings in pleasurable, affirming ways. If, however, your experiences with pornography have been negative, disturbing, pressured, or coerced, then pornography may feel like a painful or daunting topic to approach. Being aware of your own history with these materials may help you to have compassion with yourself, as well as with your child, as you navigate this complicated terrain. No matter where you're coming from, I'm confident you can find a way to engage with this important topic in a way that works for you and your family.

Parents often ask me at what age they should start talking with their child about pornography, what to say, and how to respond if or when they learn that their child has seen pornography, as well as how to mitigate potential harms or consequences. This chapter will address these and other frequently asked questions about pornography, other sexually explicit media, and how these media shape young people's sexual development. We will also examine some of the more common pornography-related problems facing teenagers and young adults, and that Kristina and Susan see in their law practice.

Note: Our focus here will be understanding developmentally typical experiences with pornography and sexually explicit media. Issues related to pornography's role in sexual abuse are beyond the scope of this book; please see "Pornography and Sexual Abuse" on page 173 for helpful resources if you are concerned about someone causing harm.

PORNOGRAPHY AND SEXUALLY EXPLICIT MEDIA

So that we're on the same page, *sexually explicit media* (SEM) is an umbrella term; it refers to all sorts of sexual media including lingerie catalogs, romance novels, photography, paintings, sculptures, animation, drawings, video games, social media memes, audio recordings, films, videos, and so on. Pornography usually refers to images, films, or videos that show clearly exposed genitals, with people engaging in various kinds of sex acts, alone or with other people. There's also *erotica*, which may be as explicit as pornography but is often created through a more artistic lens, and *obscenity*, which is sexually explicit material that is not covered under the First Amendment and is illegal to possess. However, the lines between these kinds of sexual media are blurry. Every generation has its controversies over sex-related media, whether it's Courbet's painting *L'Origine du Monde*, Anne Desclos's *Story of O*, Robert Mapplethorpe's photography, or E. L. James's *Fifty Shades of Grey*. More recently, Maia Kobabe's book *Gender Queer*—a graphic novel memoir about coming out as asexual and nonbinary—has been the subject of scrutiny and lawsuits. Where some see obscenity, others find art. US Supreme Court justice Potter Stewart's famous quote about obscenity—"I know it when I see it"—highlights the difficulty of distinguishing between these genres of expression.

Across cultures and time periods, humans have always created sexual imagery. Sculptures and paintings that show people having oral, vaginal, and anal sex—including acrobatic versions of each—have been discovered among the art and artifacts of Pompeii, Mesopotamia, ancient Greece, and Egypt. Stunning Indian temples, some more than a thousand years old, contain sculptures that depict a diverse range of human sexual behaviors. Erotic art has been discovered across multiple periods of Chinese history, including drawings, carvings, and Chinese pillow books, which provide instructive information about lovemaking. In Madagascar, I once visited a burial site with tombs beautifully adorned with paintings of people, trees, and zebu (a type of cattle), only to come across a tomb that, at each of its four corners, featured a detailed wooden sculpture of a couple engaged in intercourse.

Keeping in mind that sexual images are commonplace may offer some perspective as you're thinking about your own child encountering SEM. Most young people—across generations and cultures—have seen sexual images, including at some of the world's most famous museums. And most of the time, the sky did not fall. But just because many people have had uncomplicated experiences coming across pornography or SEM as children or teenagers does not mean that parents should ignore what their kids may see or already have seen. There's no doubt about it: Contemporary mainstream pornography depicts sex in highly aggressive ways (more so than in earlier generations of porn), with physical and verbal aggression most often targeting women. I often hear from people who describe having stumbled upon pornography as children or young teens and feeling upset or confused—even traumatized (nightmares and all)—by what they saw. Then there are the situations involving kids in early elementary school grades, whose teachers notice them attempting to act out sex acts they learned about in pornography, which they had seen during unsupervised screen time at home or on a playdate, usually unbeknownst to their parents.

Mainstream porn is also often racist, with Black women subjected to greater aggression than white women,[67] and Asian women and Black men frequently depicted in harmful, stereotypical ways.[68] If you have reason to believe that your tween or teen has seen pornography, encourage them to critically reflect on both the racist comments and the racial stereotypes that may be portrayed. Some youth, once they become aware of the persistent racism on display in many mainstream pornography videos, want nothing more to do with them. I've heard the same from some college students, too, regarding their concerns about what they perceive as unethical labor practices in pornography.

Because of how privately pornography and other SEM are often accessed today (more than 80 percent of visits are via smartphone[69]), young people often view this material when they're alone or with a friend. Thus, many parents are unaware of what their child has seen and don't have an opportunity to get them to think critically about such representations or to support them if they're feeling confused, scared, or upset about what they've seen. Being proactive about talking together about pornography and other SEM may not prevent your child from seeing it, but it can help to provider greater context and buffer them from potentially harmful consequences if or when they do.

Pornography and Sexual Abuse

It's common for young people to view SEM, whether in lingerie catalogs, on social media, or on a porn site. Usually, this is part of typical sexual development and exploration and not a major cause for concern, even though sexuality education is still needed and helps provide context. In some cases, however, older teens or adults may show pornography to kids and younger teens. Sometimes that is as far as things go; other times, showing pornography to kids is part of a pattern of sexual abuse. If you are concerned that someone you know—a friend, family member, or even your own teenager—may be behaving in inappropriate ways (or harming children), please speak up and act. The website StopItNow.org has helpful resources including guides on how to spot harmful or potentially abusive behavior and even how to file a report when warranted. By speaking up, you may be able to prevent child sexual abuse or support young people in recovering from abuse that has already happened.

MEDIA LITERACY

Unless there is an urgent need to focus on pornography (such as if your child has just come across porn and has questions about what they saw), you can start as you would with any other topic: by teaching foundational skills. Before kids learn to run, they learn to walk. And before they become critical thinkers about pornography and other SEM, it helps to first become thoughtful consumers of mainstream media such as songs, commercials, television shows, social media, and advertising. Media literacy is here to help! The National Association for Media Literacy Education defines media literacy as "the ability to access, analyze, evaluate, create, and act using all forms of communication." It's a way to help people become active, rather than passive, consumers of media and to question what they read, hear, and see. Just as talking with children about healthy friendship characteristics (feeling safe, good inside, and like they can be themselves) sets the stage for eventually discussing healthy romantic and sexual relationships, media literacy skills are foundational for later conversations about pornography and other SEM.

Kids of all ages can be taught media literacy skills. Parents and teachers can encourage them to think critically about the media around them by asking questions such as:[70]

- Who made this?
- Who is it made for?
- How does this make me feel?
- Who might be helped by this? And who might be hurt?
- Can I trust this to tell me the truth or help me in important ways?

Older children and teenagers might be encouraged to ask additional questions of the media they consume such as:

- Who profits from this?
- What does this want me to feel or do?
- What ideas, values, and points of view are shown?

- What do I understand from this and what can I learn about myself from my feelings, reactions, or interpretations?
- How are the media creators trying to keep my attention?

You can demonstrate media literacy through modeling (asking and answering your own questions) or by making a game of it within your family. Practice media literacy with shows, advertisements, songs, and social media that you like as well as those that bother you. Media literacy programs exist for elementary through college levels. Ask how your child's school incorporates media literacy into their curriculum (many already do this to some degree). The more practice your child has being a thoughtful consumer of media, the better situated they will be to ask good questions about pornography when they encounter it—not to mention mainstream media representations of dating, relationships, gender, and sexuality.

Finally, teach your child about the ways in which media creators capture and manipulate people's attention for their own profit, such as through sensational titles (called *clickbait*) and algorithms that place certain videos in the "up next" queue. On pornography websites, video titles often reinforce ideas about sex that are aggressive, misogynistic, and/or contrary to societal standards (at this writing, a popular porn site featured "Anal Slut," "How Are You This Wet, If You Don't Want It?" and "Latina Stepsisters Share Stepbrothers"*). Young people don't like to be used or manipulated. Learning how this occurs through media makes them more thoughtful consumers— or ignorers—of certain media.

---

* In recent years, "incest porn" has gotten more attention. Unfortunately, some colleagues have described seeing upticks in nonconsensual sex between stepsiblings, with some sense that there was a relationship to their viewing of pornography. We lack data on this but it feels important to mention, given what some professionals have become aware of in their communities.

MOUNTAIN OR A MOLEHILL?

When it comes to young people accessing sexual content, parents often wonder whether they are making too big of a deal over something that in reality is not so bad. Yet, decades of research shows that parents tend to underestimate kids' exposure to SEM and pornography.[71] After all, most young people view porn online through smartphones, tablets, and other devices, which make it easy to keep it out of their parents' line of sight.

Parents especially underestimate what their daughters have been exposed to as compared with their sons. Perhaps due to stereotypical ideas about boys being sex-obsessed and "good" girls being uninterested in sex, parents often cannot fathom that their daughters have seen pornography, let alone the mainstream pornography upon which tweens and teens usually stumble. In a nationally representative survey of more than three thousand teenagers and adults, only 1–4 percent of parents of teenage girls thought their daughters had seen certain types of porn, such as porn showing coercion or force. However, 10 percent of teenage girls report having already seen porn involving physical/verbal coercion or sexual force, 17 percent had come across gang bangs, one-quarter had seen double penetration, and nearly one-third had seen porn depicting facial ejaculation. Parents also underestimated their sons' exposure to certain types of pornography, but more parents guessed that their sons had seen various kinds of pornography. (Indeed, teen boys had also seen a wide range of porn, with one-third having seen gang bangs and 13 percent seeing simulated rape.)

Even if your child never watches porn, there's a good chance that their future dating and sexual partners will have seen it and may approach sex from a porn-focused lens. Some kids walk away from porn believing that sex is rough or aggressive. And viewing these images, or exploring sex with others who have, can impact a child's impressions of what kinds of sex are normative, expected, sexy, or adventurous. Watching pornography is unlikely to teach your child how to approach sex in ways that are loving, intimate, respectful, communicative, or safe.

Porn features paid adult actors following a script that is meant to arouse, entertain, and sometimes shock the viewer; it is not meant to reflect reality or to teach young people about sex. Porn also represents a narrow set of fantasies, largely marketed toward men. A good deal of the porn that is freely and easily accessible online, referred to as *mainstream porn*, falls under the category of gonzo porn, meaning it is focused almost entirely on sex acts rather than the people involved (think: lots of close-ups of genitals and sexual acts).

Thinking through what porn depicts—and what it doesn't—can help us better understand what messages it may be sending about sex to those who view it. Studies that have compared the sex acts shown in porn with the sex acts young adults report engaging in shows striking differences. Kissing and condom use tend to be underrepresented in porn, whereas anal sex and fellatio are overrepresented in porn. Cunnilingus (oral sex on a vulva/vagina) and vaginal intercourse are shown in porn at similar rates as they occur in real life. In one study that compared the sex acts depicted in more than two thousand porn videos featuring women and men with US nationally representative survey data from more than two thousand adults ages 18 through 45, there were substantial real sex/porn sex differences:[72]

- Whereas 90 percent of Americans had kissed one another during their most recent sexual experience, just 25 percent of porn scenes analyzed showed kissing.
- Although one in four young adults used a condom the last time they had sex, just 2 to 3 percent of pornographic scenes showed condom use.
- Two-thirds of women experienced orgasm the last time they had sex but women's orgasm was shown in just 12 percent of porn scenes.
- While 28 percent of adults engaged in fellatio (oral sex on a penis) the last time they had sex, 66 percent of porn scenes showed fellatio.
- Although just 4 percent of young adults had anal sex during their last sexual encounter, more than four times as many porn scenes showed anal sex between women and men.

Other studies have found that:[73]

- One-third to 88 percent of porn videos include physical aggression such as gagging, spanking, choking, slapping, and hair pulling.
- Half of mainstream porn videos include verbal aggression, such as calling someone a bitch, slut, or whore.
- In porn featuring women and men, those on the receiving end of aggression are overwhelmingly women, whereas men are usually the aggressors.
- Women in porn videos usually respond positively or neutrally to aggression, and only rarely in a negative way.
- Verbal consent communication is rare, shown in just 12 percent of scenes.
- Performers tend to be slim, and women often have breast implants, no leg/underarm/pubic hair, and small labia minora.
- Penises are average sized or larger, with ejaculation happening on command and often at far distances.

These and other studies show that mainstream porn generally depicts sex as:

- Impersonal
- Unspoken (no verbal consent)
- Unprotected (condoms are rarely used)
- Unrealistic in terms of bodies and sexual performance
- Focused on men's pleasure/orgasm more than women's pleasure/orgasm
- Rough/aggressive

If porn is a person's major source of sex information, they may view rough sex, anal sex, and fellatio as common and expected. Given how many teens first see porn as older children or young teens, many young people watch pornography for two to seven years before they have their first sexual experience with a partner. Thus, some of their formative experiences that contribute to their understanding of sex may come from pornography (and/or other SEM, including television, erotic fan fiction, and social media memes). Further, young men who are into women and whose approaches to sex are influenced by porn may be less likely to focus on women's sexual pleasure or orgasm. In one study, women said they didn't feel like their sexual pleasure mattered to a partner until they were, on average, twenty-six years old (!). To put that into perspective, these women had been having partnered sex for nearly a decade, on average, before they felt like their pleasure was prioritized. But it's not just women's partners who ignore their pleasure—young women themselves prioritize their partner's pleasure over their own, as described throughout Peggy Orenstein's book *Girls & Sex*. And in a study of Swedish teenagers, one young woman said:[74]

> *I often feel like if I have sex with a guy, I want him to have as nice a time as possible [. . .] but for me it kind of doesn't matter if I come, because I am like, "he can come, and then we can stop" . . . which is really sad because it shouldn't be that way . . . and that's probably something that may have scarred me after having watched—I mean you see it in these [porn] videos that um, you kind of do it for the guy's pleasure.*

In a study of college students' sex lives, researchers found that only 11 percent of women had an orgasm when hooking up with someone for the first time.[75] And having a second or third hookup with the same person didn't increase their odds of pleasure or orgasm all that much. In contrast, two-thirds of women having sex with a relationship partner had an orgasm. Relationship sex was rated as more pleasurable than hookups. One student described how important it was for him to give his girlfriend an orgasm, but when it came to whether women he was only hooking up with experienced orgasm, he said, "I don't give a shit." This is not an isolated example. Countless students of all genders (but more often men) describe limited investment in a casual partner's pleasure and much more interest in pleasing someone they like or love and want to see again.

People are far more likely to enjoy sex and experience orgasm with a relationship partner than a hookup. But while experiencing orgasm may be more common with relationship partners, there's no reason one cannot care about a casual partner or their pleasure. In talking with kids about sex, tell your teenager or young adult that it is important to act in ways that are caring, focused on mutual enjoyment, and attentive to their partner's needs regardless of whether they've just met the person or are in a serious relationship.

WHAT PEOPLE GET OUT OF PORN

There are many downsides to young people viewing porn, some of which are described in this chapter. But I would be remiss if I didn't describe what teenagers and young adults say about why they seek out porn and other SEM (aside from sexual arousal) and the positives they feel that they experience from watching it. (To be clear, these do not apply for younger children, just teens and young adults.) These include:

- **Understanding their attractions.** About one in six high school students identify as LGBTQ+.[76] Some young people seek out porn featuring people of different genders to learn more about the kinds of people they do (or do not) find sexually appealing.
- **Feeling represented.** Many young people intentionally seek out LGBTQ+ porn, queer feminist porn, porn featuring disabled actors, anti-racist porn, and porn featuring fat performers. Some describe how seeing people like themselves depicted as desirable and desirous human beings can feel affirming, liberating, and joyful. For some teenagers, porn is the first place they've seen kissing between two people of the same gender and that helps them feel less alone in the world.
- **Learning how sex works.** When high school sex education is offered at all, it focuses on abstinence, birth control, and STIs—not how to have sex. Yet, most teenagers and young adults engage in at least

some kind of partnered sex (hand jobs, fingering, oral sex, vaginal sex, or anal sex).[77] Like most people, young people prefer to go into new situations feeling prepared. They want to see and understand the basics of how sex works so it's not super awkward when it happens. There is an especially huge gap in sex education for LGBTQ+ youth, many of whom learn how same-sex partners make out or explore one another's bodies by watching porn.

That doesn't mean porn viewing always has the positive effects that young people expect. Some young people say they sought out porn to learn how to have sex only to end up feeling bad about their bodies because they felt they didn't measure up. Others were so shocked by the aggression they saw on screen that they became less interested in having sex in real life, either because they worried about hurting a partner or because they didn't want others to treat them that way. One gay college student told me he watched porn to learn how to have sex with other men, but unfortunately walked away with the impression that anal sex should be hard and forceful. When he took this approach with his first partner, the guy ended up feeling demeaned and degraded (not to mention in pain).

Fortunately, many young people pay attention to their own feelings and those of their partner(s) and learn from their mistakes. The young gay man listened to feedback from his partner and together they created more gentle sex that they both enjoyed. A young straight man told me about how he came to see that his expectation that partners' vulvas should be bare (hairless) was unfair and influenced by having watched porn while growing up. That the young women he hooked up with or dated during high school and college choose to keep at least some pubic hair disgusted him, even though he didn't shave his own pubic hair. Although it took him a few years, and an assertive partner who refused to shave her pubic hair to match his interests, he developed a greater appreciation for vulvas (and for women's ability to make their own choices about their bodies). And in that same Swedish study described earlier, one of the teenage girls described a shift in how she and her partner approached sex:[78]

My boyfriend and I . . . had sex in a different way when we got together,
um than we have today, and I think you can see patterns in it from porn
actually . . . like in the beginning it might have been harsher or there were
like elements of choking and . . . spanking or stuff that we later talked
about and like pointed out that "this is not normal" and like "we can't go
on like this," um, and like today it doesn't happen.

Sometimes, young people start out imitating what they learn from pornography or other SEM only to realize with time, experience, and close intimate partnerships that they get to be the authors of their own sex life. Even if your teen has unrealistic ideas about sex from having seen pornography, consider the long view. You can add complexity to their understanding of sex, giving them additional information through conversations and age-appropriate sex education materials as well as reminding them that the sex depicted in pornography is scripted, and the sex acts shown may not be safe or pleasurable in real life. They will also keep gathering information from friends, partners, and other media, and this information will help them grow their understanding of relationships and sexuality. Staying open, supportive, and askable is key, as is emphasizing the importance of creating consensual, mutually pleasurable, and joyful intimate experiences.

PORNOGRAPHY LITERACY

Cognizant of how common it is for young people to see porn, some high schools and colleges have begun to incorporate pornography literacy into school-based sex education. To be clear: These high school programs do not show pornography (which would not be acceptable to do with minors), but they do include thoughtful conversations about pornography. Pornography literacy programs focus on getting students to think critically about porn, highlighting differences between porn sex and real-life sex. They may also have as goals improving students' understandings of sexual consent and reducing dating violence. The Australian organization It's Time We Talked has a curriculum available that can be used by schools, community organizations, and families.

Even if you don't have a pornography literacy program in your community, you can still:

- **Teach your child about media literacy** so that, by the time they see pornography, they are prepared to be critical consumers of it.
- **Reinforce messages about healthy relationships.** That way, if and when your child one day sees pornography, they may reflect on whether the people they see on screen look like they're feeling safe, respected, good inside, and/or like they can be themselves.
- **Describe what pornography is and that it is meant only for adults to see.** Asking your child to look away from or to turn off pornography if they happen to find it may help delay some of their viewing until they are older and better equipped to process what they've seen and how they feel about it.

Those who like pornography might say, "But wait! Pornography is just entertainment!" And that's true. It's also true that Hollywood movies and mainstream television shows are entertainment and yet can still be problematic. Mainstream movies are equally deserving of the full media literacy treatment. But when there's so little sex education available in schools, porn often stands in. How do we know that young people learn how to have sex from watching porn? Because across many countries, that's exactly what young people say.[79] And that makes media literacy skills, along with care and intention around talking to kids about porn, so important.

What Do I Say?

Common Questions About Pornography

Q. At what age should I start talking with my kid about pornography?

For children under ten, there is not usually a reason to go into detail about pornography—especially if the family is using filters and/or settings to restrict online content, and the child's use of devices is well supervised. Even at these younger ages, however, it's a good idea for parents to let children know that the internet has some pictures and shows that are only for adults and that if they come across anything that seems scary or confusing, they should look away, turn off the device, and come talk with you. You might also establish a rule in your family that you don't look at other people's phones or devices. This can reduce the chances of them accidentally seeing pornography that a friend's older sibling may be watching when they're at a friend's house for a playdate (this happens more than I wish were the case).

If you suspect your child has seen pornography at a young age, then you may need to start these conversations earlier and revisit your family's approach to technology access and supervision.

Children tend to get more tech savvy by age ten. It's also not unusual for children between ages ten and twelve to start talking with one another about sex. If your child starts asking questions about licking or eating private areas or you find them searching on the internet for terms like "choking sex" or "rape play," then it's likely that either they or their friends have seen pornography or other SEM, or have heard about such things from other kids. As many educators say, "If they're old enough to ask the question, they're old enough to deserve an answer."

If your child is twelve or older and you haven't yet started talking about pornography, there's no time like the present. Remember: Most teens will see pornography at some point. Even if they haven't seen pornography yet, it's better for them to be prepared than caught by surprise—especially given the high likelihood that their friends and potential dating and sexual partners will have seen porn or other SEM.

Q. What should I say about pornography?

There is no one script for pornography talks. Some parents start by asking their tween or teen if they have ever heard about pornography and, if so, what they understand that to mean. Asking what they've heard from friends or kids at school can shine light on what information they may have heard as well as how they feel about what's been described to them. For children who know what sex is but don't seem to know what pornography is, you might describe it as "pictures or videos of people having sex." It's not usually necessary to go into specific details about the kinds of sex shown. Although every family is different, key messages that parents often find helpful to share include that:

- Pornography is made for adults; it is not supposed to be viewed by anyone younger than eighteen.
- Pornography is made to arouse, entertain, and even shock—but not to educate. Say that, if they have questions about bodies or sex, you're happy to talk with them. Also make sure they have access to age-appropriate books about how babies are made, puberty, and sexuality.

For teenagers, as well as older kids who you suspect may have already seen pornography or who have been asking about sexual terms, consider noting that:

- Pornography often shows aggression—especially against women (Black women in particular) and more feminine men—which is not okay.
- Pornography does not show sex the way that most people have it. Assuming this is true for you, you can say "This is not how your (father/mother) and I have sex" (this can feel reassuring if what they've seen has scared them).
- Consent conversations and condom use are rare in pornography; these are not safe approaches to sex, especially with someone a person doesn't know well.
- Women's sexual pleasure is rarely prioritized in pornography featuring women and men; stress the value of mutual pleasure, regardless of the gender(s) of those involved.
- Pornography often features racist stereotypes and racist comments.

For those going off to college, share that viewing pornography (especially when combined with masturbation) must be done discreetly. Kristina and Susan have worked on cases where students filed complaints that a roommate's viewing of pornography or other SEM made them uncomfortable in their living space.

With older teenagers and college students, consider talking about the ethical issues that have been raised in relation to some of the free mainstream porn sites. Many of my college students have expressed outrage to learn that some popular porn sites have failed to do their due diligence and have posted videos of young people that were taken or shared nonconsensually. Others have been angered to read media reports of porn actors/actresses claiming that the performers with whom they worked did things to them that were not in the script and that they did not consent to. Lately, my college students describe being concerned about the ethics and labor practices attached to the porn they consume. Accordingly, some say they've left free mainstream porn sites in search of ethically produced porn and SEM.

It can help, in these conversations, to normalize being curious about sex. Shaming kids is likely to create distance in your relationship. Say something like, "Many people your age are curious about sex, and many come across pornography, either by accident or because they wanted to see what it was all about. That's common." Share that you're concerned about them getting unrealistic impressions about what sex is like, how they deserve to be treated, and/or how to treat a partner. Whatever you talk about, try to keep an open, supportive connection between you and your child. Finally, after describing what pornography is, you might say, "If you come across something that seems like pornography, please come to me. I want to be able to talk through any questions or concerns you may have." It's even better if you can assure them that they won't get into trouble for sharing that information with you.

Q. How can I keep my child from watching pornography?

You probably cannot keep your kid from watching pornography forever, but you may be able to delay their exposure to porn until they are older and better able to make sense of what they see. Given how accessible pornography is today, most child/adolescent experts agree that it's not a matter of if a kid will see pornography but when.

Recognizing that every family is different, here are some potential approaches to delay or minimize your child's exposure to pornography. Incorporate as few or as many as fit your family.

- **Ask them not to watch porn.** This might seem basic, but many parents of older children, tweens, and teens have never even mentioned porn to their kids, hoping they haven't yet heard about it. However, the chances are high that many older children and most young teens have heard of porn and many will have already seen it. If you don't want your child to watch porn, it's okay to come out and say that, letting them know that some of the images are scary and not ones that they can just "un-see"; they may take your advice long enough to make a difference.

- **Provide alternative ways to learn about sex.** Lots of kids' early exposure to porn and/or other SEM is unintentional, resulting from searching for information on a topic about which they felt too embarrassed to ask. Being proactive about talking with children in age-appropriate ways about bodies, puberty, dating, LGBTQ+ issues, and sex may reduce some of their online searching, as can giving them age-appropriate and inclusive books. Let them know that the internet has a good deal of misinformation, as well as adult content that paints unrealistic and problematic views of sex. Say that you'd rather they start with the information you've given them and that they ask you or another trusted adult when they have questions.

- **Use filters and device settings.** Some families apply filters to their home wireless network. You can also use apps to filter each device your child might use and/or to enable Google SafeSearch. For iOS devices, parents can use Content & Privacy Restrictions to restrict access to certain apps and features or to block explicit content. Do this by going to Settings > Screen Time > Content & Privacy Restrictions > Content Restrictions. From there, you can make individualized choices related to explicit music, videos, movie ratings, and web content.

- **Remove potentially problematic apps from household phones.** You and other family members might review what's on your phones and how comfortable you'd be if your child accessed your phone. They may see sexual content on social media sites like Twitter and TikTok even if you don't personally follow accounts that post such content.

- **Have a shut-off time for devices.** Many families agree on a time when phones and devices are turned off, and perhaps stored in a central space. This is easier to manage with younger children and more difficult with older teens who may stay up late working on school assignments. With older teens, foster their independence by sharing your reasons for turning off phones and devices after a certain time. For many families, one of the most important reasons to have a shut-off time is to reduce distractions and help children get good sleep. Better sleep quality can help to reduce the risk of depression, anxiety, and crankiness (that's true for parents and sleep too).

- **Have open conversations with other parents.** If your child asks to go to a friend's house, talk with that parent about their approach to phones, other devices, and the internet (and filters) and share your expectations for while your child is visiting. Many young people have shared that the first time they saw pornography was at a friend's house, unbeknownst to the parents whose home it was. In many ways, it's the perfect storm: kids like to shock or impress one another, most kids these days have their own devices, and parents often (kindly) try to give kids their space, happy that their child has friends over and is having fun. Unfortunately, sometimes porn exposure happens and can upset kids. Thus, I strongly recommend open dialogue between parents.

  If you're worried that the parent hosting will take your questions personally, say something like, "Because I've heard of situations where kids have accidentally seen disturbing online content at one another's houses, even just accidentally, I wanted to ask you how your family plans to approach devices and internet access during the sleepover." If you are not comfortable with another family's approach to screens, it's fair to keep your child home, suggest an alternative (maybe their friend can come to your house, or you can meet at the park or a mall?), or pick up your child before bedtime in the case of a sleepover party.

- **Set the tone and the rules.** If you are hosting your child's friends at your house, take extra care to reduce exposure to porn in your home. You don't want to be the one fielding calls from upset parents in the weeks that follow. You might tell families that you have a rule about shut-off times for phones and devices or that you'll be collecting devices by a certain time. Or you can ask parents not to send their kids to your house with a phone or device, instead giving them your phone number in case they need anything while their children are at your home. If your child and their friends are teenagers, you could be direct with them about your family's rules (no watching pornography in your home, no giving out the Wi-Fi password, etc.).

- **Block internet access if you suspect any viewing of illegal SEM.** Kristina and Susan have worked on cases where there was illegal viewing of child sexual abuse materials by teenagers or young adult children in the home. If you suspect your child is engaging in illegal activity, seek professional advice and do what you can to lock down internet access. You might take away all devices (phones, computers) except for times when your child is doing homework in the presence of an adult. Then, when the homework is done, the devices are given back. Or consider password protecting internet access in your home and not freely giving out the password to your children (or their friends who come over and may want to connect their devices to the home Wi-Fi).

- **Adult supervision.** For families with young children, parents often have a rule that a parent or other trusted adult (grandparent, sitter) has to be in the same room whenever their child is using a phone, tablet, or other device. For families with older kids and teenagers (many of whom need to use devices and the internet for homework), some families say that, if they are using the device in their own room, then the door needs to be open. That said, depending on the age of an older teenager and how comfortable parents feel with sexuality, some parents may simply give their teen space, recognizing that teens need privacy not just for homework but for sexual exploration, including masturbation, and accepting that they may find a way around filters to watch pornography, even if asked not to. Parents can't control everything—and most don't want to, anyway.

Every family is different. Some boundaries are more appropriate for younger kids than older kids. Some get complicated with big families whose children span a variety of ages. What's important is that you consider your own family and its values, how long you want to try to delay access to pornography, and your child's particular needs. Some kids are prone to anxiety or nightmares over disturbing ideas or images, whether from mature music lyrics, literary themes, or movies. Others take a lot in and feel fine. Also, parents who live apart may have different rules in each household and those differences can be challenging to navigate. Many parents depend on family or neighbors for childcare and find it difficult to manage potential exposures at other people's homes.

At some point, your child will likely see pornography—either accidentally or on purpose. Try not to be too hard on them—or yourself. There's still so much you can do to support them and their sexual development.

Sexually Explicit Cartoons and Animated Images

Occasionally I hear from parents who are concerned that their teenager may be viewing *hentai,* which refers to sexually explicit anime or cartoon images (these are not the same as other forms of non-explicit anime, which is popular among young people). Viewing or possessing hentai and other similar images (*lolicon,* which depicts underage girls, and *shotacon,* which depicts underage boys) is illegal in some countries and may even be considered child sexual abuse materials. Even though these illustrated images don't involve harm to real children, some lawmakers have expressed concern that viewing such images might normalize sexual contact with children, or make it more likely for a person to sexually abuse a child or to transition into watching child sexual abuse materials. Make sure your child knows that these kinds of media are off-limits and may be illegal.

In the college context, Kristina and Susan have worked on cases where sharing hentai was evaluated as to whether the exchange was sexual harassment. While the person sending the images might consider them to be funny, the person receiving them may be uncomfortable and or feel distressed at having seen the images (especially if they were victims of child sexual abuse). Likewise, repeatedly sending sexual images of any kind may be considered harassment or stalking, as it can be construed as repeatedly making sexual overtures and advances to another person.

Q. How should I respond if I find out my child has been watching pornography?

Your response will vary based on your child's age, what kind of content they've been watching, and how often they've been watching it. Above all, take some time, try to stay calm, and remember that it's normal for kids to be curious about sex. No one wants to be shamed for wanting to learn about sexuality or for what they find sexually exciting or arousing. Having a parent walk in on them watching porn or confront them with their web browsing history can make kids feel vulnerable and shut down communication completely.

If you have walked in on your teenager watching pornography and masturbating, walk out of the room, close the door, and ask them to come and talk with you later on. Their privacy—and probably your and their need to recover from an awkward moment—trumps the need to talk that very second. When you do talk, try to approach the conversation without blame. Depending on how you discovered they had seen pornography, you might say one or more of these:

- "As we've agreed, I regularly check our family's web browsing, and it looks like you've been visiting pornography websites."
- "I want to talk about what you've seen. I'd like to hear about any questions you have for me and also share some thoughts I have."
- "You may have seen something that was upsetting, confusing, or made you have feelings you're not sure what to do with. There are some things I want you to know."
- "I want to apologize for walking into your room without knocking. I respect your privacy. However, I was surprised to see that you were watching pornography—which is not for people your age—and I hope we can talk about that choice."

- "I support your sexual curiosity as well as your right to explore your sexuality. I also understand that many kids your age have seen, or will see, pornography. Can you tell me more about how you learned about pornography and what you think of it?"

If your child seems resistant to talk, say, "We only have to talk about this for two minutes and then we can move on, if you like. Or we can keep talking; it'll be your choice." Share your thoughts and talk through your family's values, especially if you have concerns about the messages that mainstream pornography tends to send—that it can be aggressive or present harmful or unrealistic ideas about sex. Make space to hear about your teen's perspective and if there is more that you can do to support them with any questions they have about bodies or sexuality.

Q. My teen has already seen pornography. Is this going to cause problems for them later on with sex or relationships?

Most teenagers watch pornography at some point. The mere act of having seen pornography is unlikely to cause harm for them later on. However, more frequent pornography viewing may contribute to unrealistic expectations for sex, which could contribute to awkward, problematic, or (less often) even illegal behaviors. Parents can help by:

- Being askable;
- Talking about media literacy and, when a child is old enough, pornography literacy;
- Sharing that pornography is not realistic and why it should not be used as a road map for real-life sex;
- Providing fact-based information about sex, gender, and bodies (through conversations as well as age-appropriate books and websites);
- Emphasizing the importance of sexual consent, mutual pleasure, safer sex (condoms, birth control), and healthy relationships.

If we provide diverse views of sex—including those related to intimacy, affection, pleasure, communication, joy, and other ideas that are important to you—kids will have more than enough options to consider. Pornography is a common part of young people's media diet; when it's the primary source of sexual education or sexual modeling, that's when there may be more difficulties.

Even though I work on a college campus and Kristina and Susan represent students involved in sexual misconduct and assault cases, we see similar patterns in how pornography influences young people's sexual lives. Two of the more common problems we see involve nonconsensual anal sex and nonconsensual rough sex. We've dedicated the entire next chapter to some of the challenges with rough sex, but first we need to take a moment to talk about anal sex.

WHAT'S UP WITH ANAL SEX?

Anal sex between women and men has increased substantially over the past twenty-five years, and its overrepresentation in pornography has led many of my college students to describe feeling like it's something that people are supposed to try. These days, nearly half of young adults have tried anal sex at least once, although most heterosexual people who have tried it tend to engage in it only rarely (once or twice a year, if that).[80] Moreover, most straight people don't actually enjoy anal sex. Just one in three men and 14 percent of adult women say they find anal sex appealing.[81] Women often describe feeling pressured or coerced to have anal sex or that they need to have anal sex to keep their partner interested or faithful.[82] Most young women who have had anal sex describe it as painful.[83] That's not to say that no one likes anal sex—clearly some people do, especially with a partner they trust, who approaches anal penetration in a way that feels good to them, and when they start slowly or use lubricant to increase comfort and pleasure. However, anal intercourse should not be sprung on people without prior discussion. Nor should anyone ever be pressured to have anal sex (the same way they should not be pressured to have any other kind of sex). Yet far too many men—especially younger, less experienced men—do each of these, both to female and male partners.

Kristina and Susan had a case involving two college students, Cayden and Hailey, where Hailey had filed a report claiming nonconsensual anal intercourse. One afternoon, Hailey had visited Cayden at his house. After an hour of Netflix, they began sexual activity. After several minutes of vaginal intercourse, Hailey moved to her hands and knees. In the process of attempting to engage in rear-entry sex (doggy style) with Hailey, Cayden briefly penetrated Hailey's anus. Cayden claimed that he found it difficult to navigate Hailey's body and ended up in the "wrong hole." Hailey was upset with Cayden about his supposed "error"; the sudden anal penetration was not what Hailey wanted, consented to, or anticipated. When she winced, Cayden pulled out and returned to vaginal sex. Although Cayden drove Hailey home, they kissed goodbye, and they discussed plans to go out again, Hailey wanted nothing more to do with Cayden.* The next day, Hailey filed a sexual misconduct complaint against him at their university.

Whether or not it was a true mistake, we will never know. Mistakes do sometimes happen, especially with people who are new to sex. But it's also true that about one in four college men say that the way they "get" anal sex is by putting their penis into their partner's anus without asking.[84] The frequency of this strategy is confirmed by women as well as gay and bisexual men, many of whom report that a partner has attempted anal sex without first asking or discussing.[85] (To be clear: penetrating a partner without consent is not sex but assault.)

Among gay and bisexual men, some erroneously assume that everyone likes and wants anal sex and is either a top (someone who prefers to perform anal sex), a bottom (someone who prefers to receive anal sex), or versatile (can go either way). This faulty assumption leads some men to attempt anal penetration without first communicating about it. Some men just aren't into anal sex at all, what sex therapist Dr. Joe Kort has described as being a "side"

---

* In the aftermath of an assault, it's not unusual for survivors to act "normal," as if everything is okay, even if they feel violated. Some people do this because they're in shock or still processing; others are simply trying to exit a situation safely.

(rather than a top or bottom).[86] Asking "What are you into?" rather than assuming is necessary for consensual, pleasurable sex.

Kristina and Susan have seen many cases where a drunk man put his penis into someone's anus without first asking or talking about it, leading to feelings of betrayal and even physical injury. They have had cases involving two men as well as cases involving women and men. One case involved Adam, a college student who battled alcoholism. When drunk, he was mean and aggressive. Despite women ending their friendships with him and telling other women not to date him, Adam kept getting drunk and treating women in an aggressive manner. Claire was one of Adam's closest friends at college. One night, Claire asked Adam to be her date to a formal. They went to the formal for a few hours and then returned to campus. Adam invited Claire to go to another party with him at an off-campus house. At the party, Adam began to binge drink. Eventually, he was so drunk that he collapsed facedown. With the help of friends, Claire managed to get Adam back to his dorm room, where he passed out on a futon. Worried about Adam's safety, Claire stayed the night to make sure he would be okay.

Adam had no memory of what happened after passing out. Claire said that Adam invited her onto the futon to cuddle, and from there, forced himself on her, putting multiple fingers in her anus and forcing her to masturbate him. Claire ran to the bathroom and discovered that she was injured and had rectal bleeding. After Claire filed a police report and a campus sexual misconduct complaint, Adam was charged with rape. In the end, Adam pled guilty to a reduced charge and served six months in prison. Claire testified at his sentencing hearing that she had to battle ongoing post-traumatic stress disorder, making it difficult to get up in the morning and lead the life that a college student should be able to live. During the year that it took for the case to work its way through the court system, Adam entered an alcohol rehabilitation facility. He gained sobriety and a new perspective about his life and past behaviors, expressing feelings of remorse, shame, and embarrassment.

For Claire, the humiliation of being violated was difficult to discuss. When sharing the deeply personal details about what happened with Adam, Claire's tone markedly changed when she moved from discussing the consensual vaginal intercourse she had had with Adam on previous occasions to the anal penetration and excruciating pain she experienced that night. She described how violated she felt by Adam when his fingers entered her anus.

Due to the too-many-to-count instances we have seen where young people (especially women) have described feeling pressured, coerced, guilted, nagged, tricked, or forced into anal sex, we believe people who are relatively new to sex are better off exploring in physically safer and more comfortable ways. One day, they may want to try anal sex. If and when that day comes, they will likely have a more pleasurable experience if they feel comfortable with their partner, start slow, use lubricant, and explore in ways that feel good (and, of course, use a condom and discuss STI status, as described in Chapter 3).

While anal sex is a pleasurable form of sex for many people of all genders and sexual orientations, it's still advanced sex that requires greater levels of communication between partners. For young people who are relatively new to sex, it is not well suited for casual hookups. Among young gay and bisexual men, mutual masturbation and oral sex tend to be more common and are safer bets until people know one another better and feel comfortable asserting sexual boundaries and preferences (such as preferring a certain intensity of anal sex, or preferring no anal at all). No matter your teen's gender or sexual orientation, make sure to talk with them about anal sex or at least make sure that the inclusive books you've chosen for them address this important issue.

Collective Wisdom

Because older children and teenagers commonly view pornography—often for years before they ever start dating or hooking up with others—it's critical for parents to talk with their child about this important topic. Here are some key takeaways when it comes to these talks:

1. **There are good reasons to try to delay your child's exposure to pornography.** First, pornography tends to paint vastly inaccurate views of sexuality, making it seem like sex is impersonal and unprotected, and that most people (especially girls/women) want rough sex. Second, young people benefit from a chance to discover their own feelings of sexual arousal and fantasy and to imagine a sex life that *they* might enjoy—not one scripted by profit-driven producers of pornography. Third, early exposure to pornography sometimes inspires kids to mimic things they've seen, which can cause harm to peers, fractured friendships, and sometimes lead to disciplinary action at school. Through a combination of content settings, filters, technology rules, and open conversations about devices and supervision with parents of friends, there's a good chance you can delay exposure.

2. **Parents cannot bury their heads in the sand.** Pornography is easily accessible. Although families can delay pornography exposure, most teens (and many tweens) will see it at some point. Ongoing family conversations about sex, gender, consent, communication, relationships, technology, and media literacy matter.

3. **Your family's supply of age-appropriate sex education books should be kept updated.** The books that helped your young child figure out sperm, egg, and body boundaries are not the same books they need to prepare for puberty, nor are puberty books the ones to help them navigate pornography, dating, and sexual decision-making. Just as parents need to keep up with kids' ever-expanding shoe sizes, they must also keep in mind the changing sex education needs for their child's age and stage (see **Resources**).

4. **Young people are best helped by sex education that reflects their actual lives.** Many schools don't teach about anal sex (even though it's something many teens and young adults consider trying or pressure others to

try) or pornography (even though most middle and high school students have seen it). Increasingly, some parents and youth organizations are asking high schools to address pornography literacy, especially when schools give tablet computers to older kids or require them to use computers or the internet for school assignments. Supporting local, state, and school board representatives who value comprehensive sexuality education can make a difference in young people's lives and safety.

7

The Rise of Rough Sex

We're about to move into some tricky territory, including information that may feel shocking, worrisome, or scary at times. Kristina, Susan, and I had similar reactions when we first began to understand how radically sex had changed for young people and the dangers some of these changes posed, including the potential for harming oneself or others. And yet, I cannot emphasize enough how important the information in this chapter is for today's parents and caregivers of tweens, teens, and young adults. Even if you feel uncomfortable reading what follows, and even if you find yourself thinking *This can't be true*, please keep reading. The goal is to prepare and support you as a parent, even when the topics are difficult. So, deep breaths! Here we go.

One of the most profound changes to young people's sexual lives has been the recent mainstreaming of rough sex. There are many sexual practices that fall under the umbrella of rough sex and these have shifted over time. For most adults, the term *rough sex* may conjure ideas of light spanking or vigorous sex. Many have tried (and often enjoyed) sex that feels a little adventurous and maybe even kinky. Thus, some may shrug their shoulders when they hear that rough sex is now common among young people. Those of you who have come to terms with your teen or young adult child being sexually active might even be thinking: *Who cares about a little light spanking if everyone involved wants it?* Point taken. However, today's version of rough sex is different. Not only are more teenagers and young adults engaging in rough sex, but the sex itself is often more aggressive and riskier than in earlier generations. And I don't mean this in a sex-panic, pearl-clutching way; even the most sexually open-minded, kink-affirming adults I know are surprised and concerned to hear about the new sexual norms among teenagers and young adults. To complicate matters even more, today's rough sex often happens with little or no communication between partners.

Doctors, nurses, counselors, and sexual-violence prevention specialists around the world have noticed similar trends. I've been contacted by youth workers, therapists, college administrators, and attorneys from throughout the US and internationally who find themselves in unfamiliar territory, grappling with increases in rough sex situations gone wrong. Similarly, Kristina and Susan are often contacted by parents whose teens or young adult children are involved in sexual misconduct or sexual assault cases that center around rough sex practices. Often these cases involve sexual situations that started out as consensual but then one person hit, choked, or smothered the other without clear consent or prior conversation. Or, both people agreed to rough sex, but one person reported that the rough sex exceeded their agreed-upon boundaries, with them being slapped too hard or too many times, choked unconscious (instead of choked lightly), or tied to a bed and left alone.

If your heart is racing just reading this, I understand. When I share information with parents about how common and normative rough sex has become among young people today, some parents are skeptical, others are horrified, and some say "What?!? That's not normal!" In response, I encourage them to ask their teenager or young adult child what they've heard about rough sex, or specific forms of it like choking and slapping, and if people they know have tried it. In nearly every case, the parents later tell me that their teen or young adult not only confirmed that rough sex has become mainstream, but was fairly nonchalant about it, as in "Yeah, everyone chokes, what's the big deal?"

Globally, sex has changed for young people, and we need to talk about it. As you can imagine, most high schools are unlikely to teach teenagers about navigating this sensitive terrain, which leaves parents (once again!) as their child's primary sex educators. This chapter will give you a place to start. Having spent the last several years interviewing dozens of young adults who have engaged in rough sex, surveying thousands more, and reviewing the online media through which young people learn about rough sex, I've highlighted what you must know in order to navigate this topic within your own family.

If the topic of rough sex feels too daunting to address through conversation, place a sticky note in this chapter and share it with your teen or young adult. But whatever you do, don't ignore it. Many teens have already heard of rough sex (and may even have tried it), even if they're just at the stage of kissing and making out. That's right: At both the high school and college level (and sometimes even in middle school), many young people now describe being choked or slapped as part of make-out sessions. Thus, you're unlikely to risk exposing your teen to ideas they haven't yet heard of by addressing rough sex, especially if there's reason to believe they've already seen pornography. And if they haven't yet heard of it, you might want to be the first one to describe it to them so that, when they do come across it, they will be prepared, and so that their understanding of what they see or hear will be informed by more accurate information as well as your family's values.

When I've asked my college students whether and when young people should start learning fact-based information about choking and rough sex, including the risks related to these activities, they overwhelmingly suggest somewhere between eighth and tenth grade. One even said, "If you wait until tenth grade, it's too late." It's better to connect with teens earlier so that they can create safer, consensual approaches to their intimate lives.

WHAT'S CHANGED ABOUT ROUGH SEX

Because contemporary media has a global reach, with people in different countries connected through social media and often watching similar pornography, sexual norms now shift rapidly around the world. In the US, college administrators working in many states have shared that they've seen increases in sexual assault reports involving rough sex, and especially choking. Often, the young people involved consented to hooking up but did not discuss rough sex before doing it. They may have started kissing and making out and then one person started choking the other, without asking first. In Sweden, women's healthcare providers have described seeing more young women presenting at clinics with injuries from rough sex, prompting updates to sex education.[87] Responding to an uptick in rough sex–related sexual assaults, New Zealand youth workers have created educational materials to teach young people about rough sex and how to understand (and reduce) the risks. Faced with teenagers' questions about choking, Icelandic sex educators have been debating at what age to begin talking with young people about such sensitive topics.[88] And in Mozambique (as in other countries), young people describe learning about rough sex from watching pornography.[89]

As a long-time advocate of sexual pleasure and exploration, I'm not here to shame anyone for diverse forms of consensual sexual expression. Most people have tried some kind of kinky sex, even if they don't think of it that way. Also, kink and rough sex are part of a rich history of sexual liberation, especially for LGBTQ+ people who have risked a great deal to create safe spaces in which they can explore their own sexualities and push back against heteronormative ideas of sex.[90] Women of all ages and sexual orientations have also found meaning in expressing their sexuality in diverse ways, including through rough sex. But we should pay close attention when rough sex becomes a norm or expectation (especially for teenagers and young adults), with young women and LGBTQ+ youth most often at the receiving end of being choked, slapped, punched, or hit. If being choked or smothered are so great, why aren't more straight men seeking out these experiences?

Although rough sex practices have been described in art and literature for hundreds of years (think, for example, of the Marquis de Sade, *Story of O*, and—more recently—*Fifty Shades of Grey*), they were usually engaged in by only a small percentage of people, who were often connected to a kink or BDSM community. The people choosing these kinds of sex tended to be sexually experienced adults who had built sufficient trust with their partner, communicated about limits and boundaries, established safe words and/or safe gestures, and approached diverse forms of sexual expression with the care and preparation they deserve (including not using alcohol or other substances while engaged in risky forms of sex). They may have even gone to a kink or BDSM workshop or connected with people in the community to learn how to approach riskier forms of sex with communication, care, and safety in mind. This stands in stark contrast to seventeen-year-olds learning about choking and slapping through TikTok videos or Twitter memes and trying it out with someone they just met. Because conversations about whether one feels ready for sex or wants to use a condom are intimidating enough for teens just beginning to explore partnered sex, one can only imagine how ill-equipped many young people are for thoughtful conversations about being hit or choked in the name of pleasure. To be clear: often things go fine, and the sex feels good to everyone involved. But as my students sometimes describe (and Kristina and Susan's cases affirm), things can go sideways very quickly. You don't want your child to be one of these cases. It's for these reasons that many of us are concerned—not because young people are exploring their sexuality, which is a normal part of adolescence and early adulthood, even if it makes parents feel uncomfortable. (That, too, is normal.)

Some rough sex practices—even high-risk ones like choking—have become so mainstream that people feel their partners expect them to engage in them or they'll be considered boring in bed. Yet, the decision to engage in rough sex should not be made lightly and no one should assume their partner is okay with it without discussing it first. Even among more sexually experienced adults, sometimes people cross boundaries, make mistakes, emotionally and/or physically hurt someone, and (very rarely) people die. Young people often get misinformation about rough sex from their peers, partners, pornography, and social media, and this misinformation sometimes leads to uncomfortable or scary things happening—and even to injury and sexual assault. It doesn't have to be this way. As parents, we can step into the conversation, share accurate information with our kids, and encourage them to think critically and thoughtfully about these shifts in sexual behavior, as well as the kind of partner they want to be.

WHAT IS ROUGH SEX?

The term *rough sex* means different things to different people. Some of it is generational. Around 2010 (the earliest year we have data from), rough sex was largely understood by young people to mean light spanking or vigorous sex. These days, when someone says they're into rough sex, they're often talking about choking, face slapping, smothering, name-calling, or consensual nonconsensual sex (also called CNC; more on that later). How people define rough sex can also vary by gender. In studies where young adults have been asked to describe what they considered rough sex, women have offered examples like anal sex, paddling, and name-calling. In contrast, men's examples are often more extreme, including anal fisting, ball busting (hitting, punching, or kicking the testicles), urinating on a partner, or double penetration.[91]

Why does it matter what people consider rough sex? Because few people—especially those who are new to sex—are comfortable enough to have detailed conversations about even more conventional kinds of sex, let alone rough sex. They may lack experience sharing what they want to do (or not do) in real life or—in the case of rough sex—describing how hard or soft they want to be slapped or choked. Consequently, if two people are texting or talking and say that they're "into rough sex," they may walk away from that exchange with vastly different understandings about what that means. While both people may think that means hair pulling and vigorous sex are on the table, one of them may feel shocked if the other person slaps them across the face or chokes them during sex—especially if they are simultaneously being called a name like "bitch" or "whore" (since name-calling is sometimes part of rough sex). Unfortunately, these are the kinds of sexual situations that Kristina, Susan, and I hear about with regularity. And as a parent, you need to hear this so that you can have informed conversations with your child and, if they've been harmed, offer your support.

We also hear from young people who describe feeling pressured to engage in rough sex but agree anyway. Sometimes the pressure comes directly from their partner; other times, their partner isn't pressuring them but they have a sense that they "should" be into rough sex because their friends are. Also, young people don't always know how to express to their partner that they're not into rough sex. As either the giver or receiver, they may go along with the hits, slaps, chokes, or name-calling because they don't know what to do and are just trying to get out of the situation without experiencing, or causing, further harm.

Without explicit, open conversations about sex, young people often assume too much. A best-case scenario is that the misunderstanding prompts those involved to talk about sex and what they're into or not into, and then start over with better communication and clear consent, sticking only to the agreed-upon kinds of sex. I've interviewed many young people who describe successfully navigating such situations, especially if their partner is someone with whom they're in a loving, trusting relationship. Worst-case scenarios often involve injury or (in rare but tragic cases) death. My college students are often surprised to hear that the person who enacted the rough sex may find themselves facing allegations of sexual assault, rape, or even murder (if they unintentionally kill their partner such as while choking or smothering them), even if the rough sex was consensual. Let your child know that just because rough sex is consensual does not mean that they can do whatever they want to another person without consequence. Also, say that if a partner asks them to do something that is high risk or dangerous, they can (and should) say no.

Before we go any further, let's go over some forms of rough sex that have become popularized so that we're all on the same page:

- **Choking** involves using one or both hands, a forearm, or ligature (such as a belt or tie) to press against or squeeze someone's neck during sex. Because it involves external pressure to the neck (rather than internal blockage of the airways), it is technically a form of strangulation, even though most people call it choking.*
- **Face-fucking** (also called skull-fucking†) refers to aggressive fellatio or forcefully thrusting one's penis into a partner's mouth.
- **Facial ejaculation** is what it sounds like—ejaculating on a partner's face.
- **Gagging** involves thrusting one's fingers or penis down a partner's throat, sometimes to the point of the person vomiting (this is even a subgenre of porn).
- **Name-calling** involves calling one's partner names like *bitch*, *slut*, *whore*, or *fag*.
- **Punching** refers to using a closed fist to strike a partner's head, torso, or genitals.

---

* Some of Kristina and Susan's clients have drawn an (inaccurate) distinction between choking and strangulation, saying that choking refers to pressing against the sides of the throat whereas strangulation refers to pressing against the front of the throat. One young man I spoke with felt that choking was light pressure and strangulation was hard pressure. Neither of these are true; it is all strangulation and may cause injury or death.

† If you overhear your teen refer to skull-fucking or come across online searches or texts where they use sexual terms like fucking someone's brains out or describing vulvas in derogatory terms (axe wound, cum dumpster), consider engaging them in a conversation about what they make of so many terms related to sex (and vulvas) being violent. See "Standing Up Against Misogyny" (page 149).

- **Restraint** includes tying someone up (such as with a scarf or tie), engaging in rope play, or binding a partner's hands or legs with duct tape.
- **Slapping** refers to using an open hand to slap someone on the face, torso, or genitals. When done to the genitals, it may be called *pussy torture* or *penis (dick) torture*.
- **Smothering** involves placing something (often a pillow, hand, or clothing) over a partner's nose and mouth to restrict their breathing.
- **Spanking** involves using an open hand to slap a partner's butt. It can be light or hard, with hard usually meaning hard enough to leave a mark such as a bruise.

Finally, there's consensual nonconsent (CNC), which may involve people consensually role-playing a rape scenario, often incorporating various rough sex acts. The key word is *consensual*; those involved should talk ahead of time and clearly communicate about and agree on limits, boundaries, safe words, and/or safe gestures. There are countless other forms of rough sex, but these are the ones I hear about most often from my students and research participants. None of these involve expensive equipment, making them within reach for teenagers and young adults.

HOW COMMON IS ROUGH SEX?

About 80 percent of young adults, including college students, have engaged in some form of rough sex. However, because rough sex means different things to different people, let's look at some examples. In a 2020 campus-representative survey of nearly five thousand college students, some of the more common rough sex behaviors that students had engaged in were:[92]

- Being lightly spanked, reported by 86 percent of women, 40 percent of men, and 77 percent of gender-diverse students.
- Being spanked hard enough to leave a mark, reported by 55 percent of women, 16 percent of men, and 51 percent of trans/nonbinary students.

- Being choked, reported by 58 percent of women, 26 percent of men, and 45 percent of gender-diverse students. About one-quarter of these students were first choked during sexual activities when they were between ages twelve and seventeen.

Although less common, about one in ten college students have slapped a partner during sexual activities, and similar proportions have engaged in CNC. However, rough sex is not just a college-student phenomenon. Even in large US nationally representative surveys of thousands of adults, there is evidence of rough sex having become mainstream for young adults. Though it can be difficult for many parents to wrap their minds around, choking has become almost as common as vibrator use, with one in three young women reporting that they were choked during the most recent time they hooked up or had sex with someone. And genital slapping (hitting the vulva, penis, or scrotum) is reported by more than 10 percent of young adults of all genders.

Then there are the teenagers. Among fourteen- to seventeen-year-olds, about 10 percent report having choked or been choked, having slapped or been slapped (whether on the face or genitals), or engaged in name-calling. Some have even punched their partner as part of sex. Most of these rough sex experiences are described as consensual, but some are not.

HOW DO YOUNG PEOPLE LEARN ABOUT ROUGH SEX?

We expect for sexual norms to change over time. However, the mainstreaming of rough sex is not a subtle shift, but a sea change. Where did it come from? And how is it that choking/strangulation—one of the most common ways that men murder women throughout the world—is now not only prevalent among young people, but also asked for, eroticized, and enjoyed by some teenagers and sizable proportions of young adults?

In studies, young people describe learning about rough sex from pornography, friends, partners, social media, and mainstream media. *Cosmopolitan*, *Glamour*, *Men's Health*, and *Women's Health* have all featured how-to articles about rough sex. To understand what your teen or young adult child may have been exposed to, search the internet with terms like "how to choke during sex" or "how to have rough sex" or "what is consensual nonconsent?" Most of the online articles my research team have come across have included inaccurate information, such as the idea that there is a "safe way" to choke someone; indeed, many online articles describe specific recommended techniques for choking. Searching social media hashtags like #chokemedaddy or #chokekink yields hundreds of examples. And, free porn sites host thousands of videos depicting choking, smothering, gagging, and other forms of rough sex.

Then there's television and film. In the first episode of the teen drama *Euphoria*, a young woman is choked by her partner, without him asking or them discussing first. In the Netflix series *Lovesick*, a woman jokes, "I'm very close to choking you! Not in a sexy way." *Cosmo* describes smothering as "awkward and uncomfortable for some people" and "for others, it's a sexy blast."[93] Then there's the 2019 R-rated movie *Long Shot*, in which Charlotte (played by Charlize Theron) says to Fred (played by Seth Rogen), "Slap me on my ass and then choke me a little bit." With more than eleven million views, the video for the FKA twigs song "Papi Pacify" features a man's hand around her neck throughout. Shibari rope bondage has been shown on the Netflix show *Too Hot to Handle* as well as described in *Elle*, *Cosmo*, and *Esquire*.

WHY DO YOUNG PEOPLE ENGAGE IN ROUGH SEX?

The most common reasons young people give for engaging in rough sex is because it feels kinky, sexually adventurous, or exciting. They say they do it for the novelty, not to hurt someone,[94] or because it enhances their arousal or makes orgasm easier for them or their partner. Some young people also say that having sex that feels (and is) risky highlights for them how much they trust one another and that it builds intimacy. Other times, people aren't really into rough sex but feel pressured to be up for anything, or else they worry they'll be considered undesirable to their partner or "vanilla-shamed" by their peers. Additionally, people engage in rough sex because they enjoy:

- **Power play.** Some people like to feel either dominant or submissive.
- **Physical sensations.** Light spanking offers intense sensations yet little risk other than discomfort. However, hard spanking that results in bruises has become more common among young people.
- **Euphoric sensations.** When it comes to being choked or smothered, some like the dizziness, light-headedness, and euphoric sensations that result from decreased blood flow (and thus decreased oxygen) to the brain. Yet, there's a fine line between these neurological effects and losing consciousness—a difference of just seconds of sustained pressure.
- **Seeing their body in a new way.** Although anyone may find rough or kinky sex to feel liberating (especially when done in a safe context with a trustworthy partner), disabled people sometimes say that rough sex helps them experience their bodies in new ways that they appreciate.
- **Exploring gender roles.** Some people feel like taking on dominant or submissive roles during sex helps them explore—or challenge—gender roles.

Finally, some say they try rough sex because they've heard it can help them heal from prior sexual assault experiences. Most often, I hear this described by young adults as a reason they engage in CNC (and role-playing rape scenarios, specifically), as some say choosing to do it with someone they trust lets them feel in control over something they once had no control over. Yet, some mental health professionals caution against using CNC or rough sex for healing—especially given that there are many safe, effective, and well-established forms of therapy to help people heal from trauma.

All that said, not everyone seems to have a clear reason for why they've engaged in rough sex. Some feel it's expected of them. Some do it "just because."

THE DIFFERENCE BETWEEN ROUGH SEX AND SEXUAL VIOLENCE

Consensual rough sex is not the same as intimate partner violence. And yet, there's overlap between the behaviors involved in each (choking/strangulation, hitting, punching, smothering, name-calling). Something that concerns me about the rise in rough sex, and that I don't think gets enough attention, is what young people learn when they are repeatedly subjected to rough sex acts, especially those they didn't ask for or want but have come to accept. Fear is supposed to be our ally and alert us to potential danger, so what happens to our internal compass when we keep ignoring fear and telling ourselves "It's fine"?

I've heard from many young people—most often young women—who felt frightened when a partner slapped or choked them during a sexual experience. Some wondered if they would make it out alive. And yet they often said they didn't know how to tell their partner to stop. Their partner may have asked "Is this okay?" or "Should I continue?" and often they said yes. Some describe having felt too dazed or too out of it to speak up. Others feared that telling the person to stop might make things worse. Some did ask their partner to stop, but their partner ignored them, making the sex no longer consensual.

Given how common rough sex has become—and the pressure some people feel to ignore their fear and go along with it—I sometimes wonder whether young people will grow less apt to notice when they are in an abusive relationship. After all, if being slapped, smothered, or choked/strangled is no longer a red flag (even when done harder or more aggressively than consented to), what is?

Moreover, some young people have shared with me how uncomfortable they feel when their partner asks to be hit, choked, smothered, or "pretend raped." Nori, a twenty-year-old cisgender woman dating a same-aged transgender man, said, "I'm always, like, as careful as I possibly can be while still trying to, like, use the force [in choking them] that they appreciate. 'Cause

I don't wanna hurt him; yet, choking is dangerous. And he would just like, try to make an effort to teach me how to do it the 'safe' way. Um, but it's just hard." Young men, especially, have described feeling pressured to be rough or aggressive, especially if their partner sees their roughness as a sign of masculinity. These are not easy lines to walk for young people, especially when they lack guidance or support from a trusted adult.

"WHAT ELSE DO YOU DO?"

Even if your teenager doesn't watch porn or search out rough sex in the media, their current or future partner might. I've interviewed many young women who shared that they initially learned about choking or other rough sex acts when a partner did it to them the first time they had intercourse. These are not the hookup and virginity-loss stories of earlier generations. Things have changed. Kayla, a nineteen-year-old college student, offers us a glimpse into these experiences:

> I've only had one "sexual" situation in my life and I didn't know what I was walking into. I went to the dorm of this guy who I met at a friend of mine's frat and there was just a lot of pressure for me to have sex with him. I did not and he was somewhat respectful of that but the whole thing was weird. Like, we were making out and he started choking me without asking and then asked if it was okay so I said fine, because what else do you do? And then later when I told him I didn't want to have sex and he kept saying "We could do it for real" and when I said no he started dry humping me like really hard . . . like it just felt angry and was so uncomfortable. When that was done he got up and turned the light on and as I was leaving he said, "I hope that was all okay," and I just didn't know what to say.

There's a lot to unpack here. This was Kayla's first sexual experience of any kind and yet it involved unexpected and unwanted choking; angry, uncomfortable dry humping; and repeated pressure to have intercourse despite her having said no. She said it was "fine, because what else do you do?" Stories like Kayla's are clearly not instances of people incorporating rough sex into their sexual lives in ways that support mutual pleasure or joy. Rather, these are stories of young people who feel they have no other options but to accept the hand they've been dealt.

Young people have always experienced instances of being pressured into sex they've already said no to. That's bad enough. What sets this generation apart is that the sexual pressure is no longer just for oral sex or intercourse (though that persists), but often for sex that's overlaid with forms of verbal and physical aggression that used to primarily be associated with sexual assault, rape, and intimate partner violence. Another young woman said, "My partner started saying that I was a little slut and a whore and a bunch of dirty talk, I guess you'd call it, that was making me feel bad about myself. I wanted him to stop but didn't know how to say that." Then there's Cara's story about a hookup:

> I consented to have sex, but I did not consent to being hit or choked. When I verbally stated I was not enjoying it, he did not listen. I am trained in martial arts and self-defense, so I was able to stop the choke. I later found out he went on to assault several other girls, including punching one in the back of the head and almost knocking her out.

Martial arts training shouldn't be a prerequisite for dating.

How have we gotten to a place where young people—in response to being slapped, choked, or punched during sex, especially without communication or consent—think, as Kayla did, that they should go along with it, even if they're not into it? A place where they are second-guessing, as Christine Emba describes in her book *Rethinking Sex*, their gut reaction to being "surprise-choked" during sex? Someone who is wondering if they will be hurt during sex, or who feels the need to physically defend themselves while making out, is feeling threatened. This stands in stark contrast to what psychologists describe as "healthy stress," which helps us grow and flourish (as in, the healthy stress of learning to drive or asking someone on a date).

As someone who has spent much of her career focused on studying sexual pleasure and various vibrant, connecting aspects of sexuality, I sometimes wonder if I am being overly reactive. After all, people can and do consent to rough sex just like people can and do engage in other risky forms of recreation, such as skiing, scuba diving, and rock climbing. Also, rough sex is fun for many people, and many forms of it are lower risk (light spanking, vigorous sex, hair pulling). I've interviewed plenty of young people who describe pleasurable experiences with rough sex, even if there are occasional minor hiccups (a slap that's too hard, a name they don't like being called) that they discuss with their partner before moving on. However, I also hear stories from college students these days, as more young people engage in rough sex—often without really communicating about it—that suggest that my colleagues and I are not overreacting. This is not a campaign against consensual rough sex; it is, however, a call for talking about it.

CONSENT AND PLEASURE ARE TWO-WAY STREETS

Very often, consent conversations focus on the person being penetrated (in the case of oral sex or intercourse) or on the receiving end of sex acts like slapping or punching. Yet, consent and pleasure are two-way streets. When it comes to rough sex, it's important to consider whether the person being asked to slap, spank, or choke wants to do it in the first place. They may not feel comfortable engaging in what feels like aggressive or violent acts to another person, even if their partner asks for it. Teens need to hear that they can decline to do something to their partner that feels uncomfortable or dangerous. When people set boundaries, it should go both ways: people should say what they don't want their partner to do to them and also what they are not comfortable doing to their partner.

I've heard from people (especially men) who felt afraid when they were asked by a partner to choke them during sex. One young man said:

You wouldn't point a gun at someone, like, even if it was completely unloaded . . .

Choking makes me feel that way. Like, it makes me feel like I'm hurting . . . someone I really care about and I feel like I can do "gentle sex" in a way that doesn't make me feel that way even a little.

Another man, who we'll call Luis, described choking his girlfriend even though doing so made him uncomfortable. Following her request to be choked harder than in the past, he increased pressure on her neck and she unexpectedly passed out. Even though she appeared to him to lose consciousness only briefly, the experience left him shaken. Here's how he related the experience:

So her vocality drops down, but she's still very animated during sex. And then for that to stop, for her eyes to like shut and for that to stop, I mean, it, it, it makes me stressed out even now. It was, it was scary. I, um, let go immediately, stopped the sex immediately. I stopped everything and I probably pulled out too. I'm not sure, um, because at that point I just kind of held still, just kind of looked at her, and she was back in like a second and a half, like it was, it was almost instantaneous. Um, I, and I, I cried later because of how terrified I was, but I didn't cry then because I think I was mostly concerned with making sure she was okay. Um, and she said like, "Yeah, it's fine. Here's what you did wrong." The sex was over for the night . . . but she was, she was okay. She just explained what went wrong and how just that next time [to try choke her differently], um, but she could see that I was very visibly shaken.

While some people refuse their partner's requests for certain forms of rough sex, others acquiesce. Some young men feel pressured to please their partner or to prove their masculinity. This is all the more reason to raise children to feel deeply in their gut that there is no single way to be masculine (or feminine, for that matter). If a person wants to engage in consensual rough sex with a partner who asks for it, that may work for them, though they should learn ways to reduce risk (there is no risk-free or truly "safe" way to have some kinds of rough sex). If they're not into it, though, they need to feel confident that they can say no—that they can resist being pressured to have sex that doesn't make them feel safe or good inside.

Although some people engage in slapping (and like it), others describe slapping as too aggressive or violent for their taste. When it comes to facial ejaculation, some like it and others feel disrespected. And while some people like dirty talk and name-calling, it makes others feel bad, especially if they've been belittled by family or former partners. Sexual intimacy is at its best when it feels connecting or freeing. Unless partners have discussed that they both truly like and want to engage in some form of rough sex that's new to them (and this discussion occurred well in advance of having sex, and not while under the influence of drugs or alcohol), I don't recommend it.

Finally, while mistakes happen during any kind of sex, with rough sex, the stakes can be higher. While I've spoken with many people who describe situations like Luis's story above, where he accidentally choked his partner unconscious, and the two of them talk it through and move on, Kristina, Susan, and I have all seen instances where something unexpected happens and one of the people walks away feeling betrayed, hurt, or angry. This is one reason why rough sex, when practiced at all, is better off done by people who know each other well, have a great deal of sexual experience, communicate in detailed ways, and are not using substances.

OKAY, BUT ASSUMING PEOPLE CONSENT TO ROUGH SEX, WHAT'S THE HARM?

Even when rough sex is consensual, it's important to understand some of the possible short-term and long-term consequences. There are some forms that are best avoided due to their posing a higher level of risk. Although there are unlikely to be long-term effects from lighter forms of consensual rough sex, such as light spanking, light scratching, or name-calling, some forms of rough sex can and do lead to serious injury or even death. Slaps and punches to the face or head can cause concussion or other head trauma and can burst blood vessels in the eyes, causing changes to vision. Being hit on the genitals can lead to substantial bruising. Also, some people feel scared or traumatized from nonconsensual rough sex or from rough sex that was harder or more aggressive than they anticipated. Mental health consequences matter too.

Choking is a higher risk form of sex and yet, as we've seen, it's prevalent. As any doctor, nurse, or coroner will attest, choking/strangulation can hurt and kill—even if it's done briefly or without much pressure. Although being killed while being choked during consensual sex is rare, a recent review of BDSM-related deaths found that choking/strangulation was the most common cause of death, accounting for 88 percent of cases. Because of this risk, many people who are part of kink and BDSM communities have long avoided choking/strangulation, smothering, and other forms of sex that decrease oxygen to the brain. Some BDSM clubs and spaces even ban members from engaging in such sexual practices.[95]

When I've interviewed college students about choking, many are quick to point out that the way they choke is "safe." Yet, there is no way to choke or be choked that is completely free of risk. In addition to the low but real danger of killing someone while choking them, being choked (which, again, is a form of strangulation)—especially repeatedly—may increase a person's likelihood of depression, anxiety, recurrent headaches, ringing in the ears, or even stroke.[96] There are cumulative effects on the brain when it's repeatedly deprived of oxygen and other nutrients found in blood. Up to 30 percent of young adults who have been choked during sex have experienced alterations in consciousness (dizziness, light-headedness, temporary vision changes, or loss of consciousness), which have been associated with negative long-term mental health and cognitive difficulties.[97] Further, studies find neurological differences between young women who have been choked often and those who have never been choked.[98] Let your teen or young adult know that, no matter what their friends or partners or social media videos say, choking is a higher risk activity, and they would be wise to avoid it.

When rough sex injuries do occur, people often delay or avoid seeking healthcare, well aware of social stigmas around alternative sex practices.

Those who do seek care may attempt to hide the source of their injuries from their healthcare provider, claiming they had an accident or suffered a sports injury. In one study of college students, just 1 percent of women and 7 percent of men who experienced choking-related symptoms discussed them with a nurse or doctor. While the most common reason they chose not to seek care was because the symptoms improved quickly or "didn't seem like a big deal," young women (more often than young men) said they didn't tell a healthcare provider because they worried about being judged. And, regardless of gender, students said they chose not to discuss with a provider because they worried about their parents finding out. Again, a warm and supportive parenting style cannot prevent or fix everything, but it is helpful for kids to feel like they can turn to their parents for help and support if and when things go wrong. When someone feels like their parent will shame or judge them, or come down too hard on them ("I told you never to do that!"), they may be less likely to ask their parent for help or be forthcoming with them.

In addition to harm from choking itself, healthcare visits are often expensive. Just as many parents talk with their teenagers about the risks and costs associated with driving (including risks and costs associated with car accidents), talk with your teen about the potential risks and costs associated with rough sex (and any rough sex accidents). Again, this isn't about scaring them, but if they are going to engage in rough sex, they need to consider the realities and potential consequences and then decide how to mitigate risk and be safe with their partner(s).

CAN YOU CONSENT TO ROUGH SEX IN ADVANCE?

As noted earlier, consent conversations should happen at the time of sexual activity. However, because Kristina, Susan, and I see this go wrong so often, especially when it comes to rough sex, it bears repeating in this chapter. As rough sex has become more mainstream, young people often text each other rough-sex fantasies in detail (e.g., "Choke me unconscious" or "Face-fuck me"). Sharing fantasies or desires is common, but sharing ideas over text is not the same as consent. When they get together in person, they should have clear (preferably verbal) communication before moving down the path of rough sex. And again, consent alone is not enough. Partners who are interested in each other's pleasure and enjoyment will want to establish (and revisit) not only clear consent, but also details on how, under what conditions, and what feels good.

Rough Sex and Consent

Kristina and Susan still remember their first "rough sex" case, from quite a few years back now. Andres was seeking legal representation for a campus sexual misconduct case involving serious allegations of sexual assault unlike any Kristina and Susan had previously encountered. In an extensive intake meeting, Andres described his relationship with Deja. As he discussed the flirtation and sexual events leading up to Deja's report of assault, including the various ways they had sexually explored together, Kristina and Susan tried to remain stoic. Inside, however, their reaction was shock mixed with a bit of wonderment, asking themselves, *Do people really do this stuff?*

Andres had a very matter-of-fact tone as he described his interest in BDSM (a term some people use interchangeably with kink and rough sex, even though there can be differences). Andres explained that BDSM was common among college students, and that he had engaged in many types of rough sex with prior partners. Most of the time these behaviors included choking and inflicting some sort of physical pain during sexual intercourse and had included spanking, using sex devices, and tying each other up with rope and other restraints. At a certain point in his sexual interactions with Deja, however, things went too far for Deja. She filed a campus report because she felt scared and violated.

One day after a late afternoon class, Andres and Deja had wandered into an empty classroom. They began kissing and groping, keeping their eyes and ears open for any passersby who might catch them fooling around. Both people initially described the possibility of getting caught as arousing and exciting. The sexual acts escalated and eventually, Andres leaned Deja over a desk, where he choked her, spanked her, and pulled her hair. What Andres thought was consensual and enjoyable, Deja viewed as nonconsensual and terrifying.

In reviewing hundreds of text messages and online chats between Andres and Deja, it was clear that they had spent hours discussing their mutual interest in BDSM. They had shared with one another that they enjoyed rough sex and each had significant experience with it. Eventually, Andres and Deja began to talk about becoming sexually active with one other. They even discussed the importance of safe words and agreed upon their own safe words for rough sex with one other. During their discussions (albeit only through text and online chat), they spent a lot of time anticipating how amazing the sex would be when it happened. All that was left was an opportunity for them to get together and act out what they discussed.

Andres described their first sexual encounter as "normal"; they made out and Andres performed oral sex on Deja. After oral sex, Deja asked to pause and stated she was not ready to go "all the way" (i.e., have intercourse). They continued to date, and their text messages got more explicit about BDSM and rough sex. At his campus Title IX hearing, Andres stated that after many nights of discussing their mutual interest in rough sex, he thought that Deja wanted to try some spanking and other rough sex that evening in the classroom. According to Andres, Deja never used her safe word. From his perspective, that meant things were going all right—even though it may also have meant that Deja was scared and didn't know how to ask Andres to stop.

The hearing panel quickly dismissed Andres's texts and online chats as evidence of Deja's consent to the sexual behaviors in the classroom under the reasoning that expressions of interest are not the same as in-the-moment consent. The panel concluded that Andres violated the school's

Title IX policy, which required affirmative consent. The panel expelled Andres from school.

PREVENTING UNWANTED ROUGH SEX

Ideally, people who want to incorporate rough sex into their sexual lives should talk about it before doing it and only proceed if there is clear consent to do so. However, my experience interviewing young people about their sexual lives is that some people only discuss sex ahead of time, and then shy away from sexuality-related conversations in the moment. For example, many young people describe doing something rough with a partner because "there was just this vibe" or "I could tell from their energy." Sex has a better chance of going well in terms of both consent and pleasure if people take a beat and communicate rather than guess.

In describing how common it has become for young people to initiate rough sex acts without first discussing it, some of my students shared in class that they've found it helpful to preemptively talk about rough sex, being very clear prior to or at the start of a hookup what they are or are not okay with doing. That is, as people are getting to know one another, or as they're messaging about a potential hookup or things are starting to heat up, in addition to insisting on a condom (if intercourse is on the table), people can say, "By the way, I'm not into _____ (whatever the person is not into) so please don't try it." Also, people who don't want to be rough with their partner, can say "I'm not comfortable _____ (choking, hitting, etc.) people, so please don't ask me to. I won't do it." Alternatively, they can also say what they are into and what they'd like to do with one another.

Ideally, this will stop unwanted rough sex before it starts. But even clear communication does not always work; in a March 2021 Reddit thread, a young woman wrote that she's repeatedly hooked up with men who have choked her, even after she has told them not to. Fifteen thousand responses later, the thread was full of young people feeling frustrated and angry, but far less alone in their shared experiences of nonconsensual choking. Please tell your teenager or young adult child not to be rough with someone without first discussing it with, and getting clear consent from, their partner—and to always respect a "no" or "stop." Finally, laws are changing, and in some places, even consensual choking/strangulation may be prohibited. Try to learn about laws in your area and discuss them with your teenager or young adult.

ROUGH SEX AND HARM REDUCTION

Just as there is no such thing as "safe sex" (due to the risk of pregnancy, STIs, vaginal tears, and so on), there is also no such thing as "safe rough sex." However, people can take steps to reduce the risk of serious harm to themselves or others.

No doubt some of you are thinking that teaching young people about "safer" forms of rough sex is a bridge too far. I get it. Yet, young adults have been clear: they don't want to hear "just say no" or what they describe as an abstinence approach to rough sex. Rather, they have been asking educators around the world for frank information on how they can have safer sex in a world in which rough sex is common. With that in mind, health experts—including from WebMD[99] and the New Zealand youth organization The Light Project[100]—have suggested ways to potentially reduce risk related to rough sex. People can:

- **Choose lower risk forms of sex.** This means avoiding sex acts that pose a higher risk for injury or death (choking, smothering, slaps or punches to the head), instead considering safer ways to explore such as oral sex, various intercourse positions, role-playing, spanking, or sex toy play.
- **Communicate about any new kinds of sex they may wish to try together.** People shouldn't introduce a new form of sex—whether rough or vanilla—without first discussing it while sober and giving one another plenty of time to decide.

- **Go into detail.** Discussing limits, boundaries (types of sex that are and are not okay with each person), and preferences related to pressure, intensity, and duration helps to make sure everyone is on the same page.

- **Discuss any relevant health conditions or prior traumas.** Some people with trauma histories might be comfortable being called names during sex, whereas for others that would be triggering. Also, people with histories of seizure, concussion, and/or cardiovascular conditions may be at greater risk for negative health outcomes from being choked, which decreases oxygen to the brain (though, again, people would be wise to avoid choking, full stop).

- **Learn skills and safety knowledge.** Young adults who are interested in rough sex might consider taking a class or workshop specific to their interest that focuses on consent, communication, and risk reduction. Some experts encourage seeking out training related to first aid and CPR,[101] especially if engaging in riskier forms of sex.

- **Choose (and use) safe words and/or gestures.** The stoplight system for safe words is often used because it's easy to remember: red means stop immediately, yellow may mean lighten up or proceed but more carefully, and green means "more, please!"

- **Stay sober.** Studies show that sex is more pleasurable (and more wanted) when it's done sober. Also, having sex while sober helps reduce the chances that someone will get carried away or be unaware of how their partner is feeling.

- **Care for one another.** Whether through cuddling right after, texting shortly after parting ways, or grabbing coffee/tea the next day, people should check in with one other after a sexual encounter to see how they're each feeling. Aftercare is especially important after rough sex, which can leave some people feeling especially vulnerable (or even bruised, hurt, or with marks on their body).

I've heard of enough rough-sex-gone-wrong situations to believe that young people would probably be wise to delay rough sex until they're older, more experienced, and more comfortable communicating with partners (and skipping high-risk forms of rough sex entirely). However, given the reality that many young people are already exploring rough sex, talking openly about health risks, communication, caretaking, and consent may reduce some of the potential harms.

What Do I Say?

Talking About Rough Sex

Q. When should I talk with my teenager or young adult child about rough sex?

Consider building a foundation with even young children, with age-appropriate messages you can add to when they're much older. Parents can teach their children that we have to always be able to see a baby's nose and mouth, since when we can see both parts, we know they can breathe, and that they should never press against or squeeze other people's necks while they're playing. Many of us teach this anyway, but these are the safety blocks to keep building upon, reinforcing the idea that necks are sensitive body parts with which we must be careful and that being able to breathe freely is essential for life. Parents of tweens and teens can look for opportunities to talk about choking during sex, especially when they are referenced in the media. And for parents who believe their teenager may be making out or sexually active with a partner, in addition to talking about condoms, birth control (for those with other-sex partners), and consent, they should also talk about rough sex.

Q. What should I say to my teenager or young adult child about rough sex?

If you have been building a foundation with open conversations about sexuality, then you have a place to start. Perhaps you've even told your child that you're reading this book. You might say, "I've heard that many young people are now engaging in choking during sex. Have you heard anything about that from friends or TV shows?" Parents often get more information from young people when asking about their peers or media than about their own lives.

If your child has watched *Euphoria* or read or watched *Fifty Shades of Grey*, your homework is to read or watch it too. If you've watched a show together and there's a scene that involves rough sex, use it as a conversation piece. This is an opportunity to communicate your family's values, your love for your child, and any concerns for their and their partner's safety.

Make sure your child knows that no one should engage in any kind of sex they're not into—that's true for vanilla sex as well as rough sex. Although some people genuinely enjoy rough sex, others do not want to be on either the giving or receiving end of it. That's okay. If they're worried they'll be seen as a prude or too boring, validate those feelings and also reassure them that there's nothing wrong with more conventional forms of sex. Our studies show this time and again: what tends to matter most for pleasurable sex is intimacy and connection.

If your child shares information with you about things they have heard others say about rough sex, ask, "What do you think about that?" You might also look for opportunities to discuss the potential health risks of some kinds of rough sex, including the risks for brain damage. Say, "You know, choking is actually a form of strangulation. It can hurt people and, in rare cases, even kill people. As your parent who loves you and wants you to live a long time—and not hurt people or wind up in prison—I'm going to strongly encourage you not to choke anyone and not to let anyone choke you."

Q. Are there ways of telling if my child is already engaging in rough sex?

Not usually, but sometimes. Bruising can occur from some forms of rough sex, especially those that involve pressure. Although most people don't bruise from being choked, about one in six young adults who have been choked have noticed a bruise at least once—sometimes in the form of a hand or multiple fingerprints. Other times, parents notice bruises or bite marks on the body. Don't turn a blind eye to these marks, thinking they're just "hickeys." Increasingly, college students tell me that someone has noticed a bruise or bite mark on their body and checked to make sure they are safe and not being abused. In these instances, the students have reassured their friend, roommate, parent, or healthcare provider that the mark was from a consensual sexual experience. Even if your child says it's consensual when asked, it gives you a chance to check in, talk about safety, and make sure that they are truly enjoying the sex they're having and not feeling pressured.

Most parents accept that sexual exploration is a normal part of adolescence and young adulthood. If you feel this way too, then remind your teen or young adult that you aren't trying to stand in the way of them creating mutually pleasurable, consensual experiences. Nor do you want to shame them. Rather, you care about their safety and that of their partner. Remind them that their safety is important to you, mutual consent is critical, and that you hope they will prioritize shared pleasure alongside communication, care, and respect. Talking about rough sex is necessary these days, from the perspectives of health, consent, and mutual pleasure. It may be uncomfortable, but you can do this.

Collective Wisdom

Although some young people have pleasurable, uncomplicated rough sex encounters, it's not unusual to experience some bumps along the road. Because rough sex that goes poorly can lead to people feeling scared or hurt, as well as student discipline or criminal charges, it's important to talk with your teenager or young adult in frank ways. Let them know that:

1. **They don't have to do rough things to their partner, even if their partner asks them to.** It's okay to say "I'm not comfortable doing that" or to prefer gentler kinds of sex. Even though some young people think that rough sex is the norm, research shows that more people are into gentle sex than rough sex (and many people like both).
2. **No one should feel the need to participate in specific types of sexual activity just to fit in.** We all get to create our own sexual lives and set our own boundaries.

3. **Rough sex is not for casual hookups.** As we've seen in some examples in this chapter, rough sex can be complicated and is best avoided by people who have just met or only hooked up a few times previously. Trust and familiarity make for safer situations, especially for young people who are new to sex.

4. **Rough sex should not be sprung on people.** There should be time for either person to back out without feeling guilty for changing their mind (though remember that a person can *always* change their mind, including in the middle of sex, whether vanilla or rough).

5. **If partners agree that rough sex is part of their routine and they don't wish to talk about it each and every time, they should still look for ways to reduce risk.** They should set hard limits (things that under no circumstances are okay to do) before going forward, have clear safe words/safe gestures in place, start out gently, check in often, and support one another through aftercare.

6. **They should err on the side of treating one another gently.** Too often, young people say that, although they agreed to rough sex, it ended up being harder or more harmful than they imagined (one can like being slapped yet not enjoy being walloped). These unexpectedly scary encounters can lead to injury, and also to the aggressor not having a second chance with their partner, who may write them off as too rough or "rapey." Sometimes, sexual misconduct or assault reports are filed. Until people know one another well and have developed enough comfort and confidence to truly communicate with one another about sexual likes and dislikes, it's a good idea to err on the side of being careful and gentle with one another's bodies.

7. **They should avoid higher risk forms of rough sex altogether.** With choking, smothering, or slaps or punches to the head or genitals, there is a real possibility of scaring or hurting someone, not to mention being expelled from school or incarcerated (or, in rare cases, killing someone). The world is full of safer yet pleasurable forms of sexual exploration.

8. **Alcohol and rough sex don't mix at all.** People who want to engage in rough sex must have all of their faculties about them so that they can effectively

be mindful of what is happening and the level of intensity or pressure they're using, as well as how their partner is responding.

9. **Good sex requires reflection and self-advocacy.** It's okay to say, "I know I said that I liked (insert type of sex) and I didn't tell you to stop, but after thinking about it, I don't really like that, so please don't do that to me again." Or, "I do like that, but only when you don't call me 'bitch' at the same time." Or, "I enjoy doing that together, but only when we're both sober."

Finally, try to approach the topic of rough sex in a way that does not shame or belittle your child. Keep in mind that while some young people are looking for a trusted adult to tell them it's okay to either delay or avoid rough sex, many like rough sex and most describe their experiences as consensual and pleasurable. Most young people are aware that rough sex is risky, and they want to learn to navigate it in safer ways. It's easier for kids to open up when their parent makes it clear that they will love, accept, and support them, even if they don't fully understand their choices.

8

Sex on the Spectrum

Before I began my training in sexuality research and education, I worked with children who had been diagnosed with what is now called autism spectrum disorder (ASD). In this work, I helped young children develop verbal and nonverbal language, improve social learning skills, manage anxiety, and identify their own and others' feelings. At the time, there was little known about the kinds of sexuality and relationship education needed to support autistic* kids at various ages and developmental stages. Since that

---

* Over the past few decades, there have been shifts in recommendations concerning the use of person-first language (e.g., person with ASD) versus identity-first language "autistic individuals." I have written this chapter cognizant of these shifts as well as people's own personal preferences around language. The choice to mostly use identity-first language ("autistic individual") was made to honor the language preference of many in the community for whom being autistic is an important and valued part of their identity. At times, I also use "people with ASD" because it, too, is preferred by some, and I wanted to be respectful of diverse views. Nothing is one size fits all. Some people use totally different terms (e.g., aspies, spectrumites). Use whatever feels best with your family and loved ones.

time, I've been heartened to see progress in sexuality education curricula tailored to the needs, desires, and strengths of autistic people, even though the field still has a long way to go. Similarly, there has been more research that amplifies autistic individuals' voices and perspectives, recognizing that they are the experts on their own lives and can best describe their needs, the ways they can successfully navigate sexual situations, and what can help them thrive. About one in forty-four US children are diagnosed with autism spectrum disorder, with more boys than girls receiving this diagnosis. And all children deserve to learn about their bodies, be prepared for puberty, learn about sexual feelings and behaviors, and hear from both their families and the professionals who support them that dating, relationships, and sexuality may be possibilities for them too.

With greater support available than in previous generations, many more autistic kids attend high school, enroll in college, and/or live and work independently in their community. These opportunities broaden young autistic adults' social networks as well as their romantic and sexual possibilities, making sex education all the more important. Even if your child is neurotypical, make sure you read this chapter. It is likely that some of their classmates are neurodiverse, and your teenager or young adult may date, partner with, and/or be romantically interested in an autistic person now or in the future. Autistic people have often had to devote enormous time and effort learning about neurotypical ways of thinking and being, including in sexual situations; everyone benefits when neurotypical people learn about the perspectives and needs of those on the spectrum in return.

Throughout this chapter I have drawn from diverse literature, doing my best to center the research and sex education curricula that directly engaged autistic individuals as study participants, leaders, or experts in their development. These studies are complemented by research and programs that have engaged parents of autistic individuals, recognizing that parents and caregivers tend to be the main sexuality educators of autistic kids.

Here, you will find descriptions of what autistic tweens, teens, and young adults say they need when it comes to learning about dating, relationships, bodies, and sexuality. Although these ideas emerge from autistic individuals themselves, they will not feel like a good fit for everyone, given the diversity of people on the spectrum. Take what feels like a good fit for where your child might be today, come back later for what might work when they're a bit older, and leave the rest. We approach this chapter from a place of respect, care, and recognizing difference rather than deficit. Although many of these suggestions come from autistic people themselves (including some of my former students and study participants), there are some inherent biases, as these ideas will generally reflect the opinions and ideas of a subset of autistic individuals (i.e., most often those who use some level of verbal language and who do not have an intellectual disability; about 30 percent of autistic people have been diagnosed with an intellectual disability, meaning they have an IQ of less than or equal to 70).

Kristina and Susan, whose practice includes a focus on special education issues, regularly see some of the challenges that autistic students bump up against when it comes to campus-level processes, which typically aren't designed to understand how students on the spectrum understand social cues. Their experience suggests that, in some instances, schools don't adequately take into account a student's accommodations when an autistic student has been accused of violating school policies on sexual harassment and sexual assault. It's not that sexual misconduct charges shouldn't be brought when the accused has ASD; of course, they should. However, it helps to consider a person's behavior in the larger context of who they are in order to provide appropriate education, counseling, skill development, or other services to help the person consider how their actions impacted another person and to prevent future harm.

UNDERSTANDING DIVERSITY AMONG AUTISTIC PEOPLE

Although there is a great deal of diversity among people with ASD, autistic individuals tend to share some common characteristics. They may experience challenges related to understanding nonverbal cues and nuance, sensory processing, verbal language, and/or understanding social norms largely developed and enforced by neurotypical people (e.g., how to make small talk or polite conversation). Also, some autistic individuals have certain strengths in common, especially those sometimes described as higher functioning. These may include learning information quickly, having a strong ability to memorize facts and statistics, and/or being able to understand complex topics, including scientific concepts. And what feels like a challenge to some is actually a strength and an asset to others. Clearly, we can't stereotype, and there are always exceptions, as with neurotypical people. Again, as we move through this chapter, please keep this diversity in mind; some of the ideas presented here will feel true for some autistic people and not for others. Everyone is unique.

Also, so much of how we think about one another depends on our perspective. For example, autistic people are often described as rigidly adhering to rules or sticking to black-and-white-thinking. And, when I think about the many autistic people in my life over the years, it's true that most have had rigid rules or routines (a certain order of listening to songs, lining up paper in an extraordinarily straight line, following a specific path to get to class) and that any deviation could cause substantial stress. However, it's also true that autistic people tend to be more flexible about some things, too, including ideas about gender, sexual orientation, and sexual expression. Some neurotypical people are extremely rigid in their thoughts about gender or sexual orientation, insisting on a man/woman gender binary or that only heterosexuality is natural (despite ample evidence to the contrary throughout human history) and getting stressed about people who express themselves outside these rigidly defined categories. Perspective matters.

Further, not all challenges faced by autistic people are due to ASD itself. As is true for neurotypical people, some autistic teenagers and young adults have more than one diagnosis; these comorbidities may include depression, anxiety, ADHD, obsessive-compulsive disorder, gastrointestinal (GI) issues, seizure disorder, or other physical or mental health issues. And many challenges have nothing to do with the person themself but rather with the rules, processes, and systems constructed by neurotypical people that aren't easy for autistic people to navigate.

Yet, whatever challenges a person has, and whether they are related to ASD or not, we all have sexual rights. As described by the World Association for Sexual Health, these include rights to accurate and understandable sexuality information, sexual privacy, sexual pleasure, sexual and reproductive autonomy, and living free of sexual coercion and violence. And all humans have these rights—not just neurotypical people. As such, sexuality education that is attentive to, and inclusive of, the needs and desires of autistic people is vital.

SEXUAL AND GENDER IDENTITY

A consistent finding among studies involving autistic teenagers and adults is that there is substantial diversity when it comes to how people describe their gender identity and sexual orientation.[102] It's not only that young autistic people may be more likely to identify as bisexual or gay as compared to their non-autistic peers, but that they are also more likely to identify with less common sexual identities (such as being pansexual, asexual, or sapiosexual—the latter refers to being oriented toward smart people) and gender identities (nonbinary, bigender, agender), as well as diverse relationship identities (such as being polyamorous or demiromantic). If you're not sure what your child means by their gender, sexual, and/or romantic identities, ask them. Labels change from time to time. I'm a seasoned sexuality educator, and my students still surprise me with identities that are new to me. Showing kind and sincere curiosity about your child's identity and what it means to them may help you learn more about them and their inner world and help you grow closer. It also gives you and your child practice communicating about sexual and/or romantic feelings. For example, some asexual-identified (also called "ace") people have never experienced sexual attraction to or desire to be sexual with other people, whereas others describe feeling low sexual desire or highly selective sexual desire. Some asexual people masturbate or have sex with others; some do not. Rather than assume, just ask. Also, parents need to understand that while some students are firm with their identities, others change over time (a concept called "sexual fluidity")—something that is also true for neurotypical people.

Some speculate that autistic individuals may more often identify in gender diverse and non-heterosexual ways because they don't feel the same social pressures to fit into cisgender, heterosexual norms created by neurotypical people. While growing up, autistic children may be less likely to pick up on the social cues that their neurotypical peers may notice and adhere to so that they can perform gender in ways that seem acceptable in their families or communities. It's also been suggested that autistic people are more comfortable being open about LGBTQ+ identities because they are used to being frank about many things in life and may not worry about feeling out of place to the same degree as neurotypical people, for whom being seen as "normal" often feels so important.

Why does the fact that so many autistic people identify as LGBTQ+ matter? As discussed earlier, school-based sexuality education is often focused on heterosexual experiences, such as safer sex between women and men and the kinds of sex that women and men have (prioritizing penile-vaginal intercourse). Many schools don't teach about LGBTQ+ identities or sexuality at all. Because of this, autistic tweens and teens may feel and be doubly ignored. That's not good for their mental health or physical health.

LEARNING ABOUT SEX

Young autistic people develop physically (think menstrual periods, first ejaculation, masturbation) along the same timelines as their peers. However, autistic kids' social awareness may develop in ways that make it difficult to pick up on unwritten rules created by neurotypical people, such as how to show someone that you like them or why personal hygiene matters to both friendships and making romantic and/or sexual connections. This disconnect can contribute to delays in the development of their skills related to relationships and sexual behavior.

Peer groups and other social relationships also influence what children will learn and when. Non-autistic children often complement what little sex education they receive from school with information gleaned from social sources such as friends, cousins, crushes, and dating partners. Even if their teachers and parents are tight-lipped on sexuality topics, they have a broad world from which they can learn about sex. However, autistic kids don't often have these same social connections or opportunities for social learning. Accordingly, they primarily learn about sexuality topics from their parents and other caregivers and thus generally wind up with limited knowledge about sex.

Further, many parents and caregivers find themselves needing to spend so much time and energy on teaching basic hygiene like brushing teeth or being vigilant about safety issues (like preventing their child from wandering off) that they understandably can't get to other issues. Parents being stretched too thin, with little community support, is a real issue. The idea of sitting down and engaging in a sex talk may seem like a luxury they just don't have.

Unfortunately, this lack of sex-and-dating education contributes to later problems with peers. In addition to the fact that limited sexual knowledge hampers autistic people's ability to create healthy relationships as well as safe and pleasurable sexual experiences, studies show that being less knowledgeable about sex may also increase autistic kids' vulnerability to sexual harm. The protective role of sexual knowledge applies to young people with and without ASD and is one of many reasons why body and sexuality education is so important. Although being knowledgeable about bodies and sex cannot completely protect a person from sexual abuse or assault, it can reduce risk by helping the person spot red flags.

When autistic youth do learn about sex from sources other than their parents and caregivers, they tend to turn to nonsocial sources of information such as watching television and searching the internet.[103] But it can be difficult for young people to tell which sites are trustworthy. It's helpful for parents to provide high-quality sex education books to their child, whether through offering a physical book to read, finding an audio version to share, reading out loud to them, or reading on one's own and then sharing the highlights as part of sex talks.

Many parents of autistic kids delay or avoid conversations about sexuality because they feel unsure about whether their child will ever have the opportunity for romantic or sexual relationships.[104] If your child has limited verbal abilities, you might wonder what questions are stirring inside them (unbeknownst to you) or how to address your child's basic questions on sexuality. Additionally, some parents of autistic children delay or avoid sex conversations for the same reasons parents of neurotypical children hesitate to broach the subject (feeling unsure what to say or uncomfortable talking about sex). Finally, many well-intentioned parents, educators, and healthcare providers just don't know how to have these conversations in a way that will be understood, as many of these conversations require complex communication skills. If consent is confusing for a neurotypical student, think how difficult it could be for a student who struggles with nonverbal communication. For all these reasons, many autistic teenagers and young adults describe feeling like they don't have the knowledge about sexuality or relationships that they wish they had. Below are some tips to support autistic children in learning about sex, bodies, and relationships.

What Do I Say?

Talking to Autistic Kids About Sex

Q: My child has done many things later than their peers without autism, whether talking, tying their shoes, or making their first friend. When should I start talking with them about sex?

As with any child, talk early and talk often. Most kids learn bits and pieces from these conversations and, over time, build up sufficient vocabulary, knowledge, and cognitive skills to put it all together. If your child has cognitive delays, hearing the information multiple times may help them to better understand it. Also, it's never too late to start. Autistic people often make it into adulthood with a later start on dating and sex than their neurotypical peers; this is fine if they feel comfortable with it, but some kids feel behind, especially if they perceive that people their age should be having romantic experiences.

Even if your child doesn't ask, make sure they have age-appropriate and developmentally appropriate information that's needed at each life stage. For example, young children need language for their body parts, including their genitals, as well as rules about who should or should not be touching those parts; older children need information about puberty, periods, pubic hair, erections, wet dreams, increased sweating, vaginal discharge, body odor, and other pubertal changes. Teenagers and young adults need information about sexual feelings and behaviors, safer sex, and relationships. This is not an exhaustive list; I've provided examples of developmental needs throughout this book as well as suggestions for books and websites in **Resources**.

Q: My child has caregivers who work on a lot of different life skills. Is it fair to ask them to help out with sex education too?
Absolutely! It depends on their background, training, and comfort level, of course, but if your child has caregivers who could support them in this area, it's fair to ask them. Some recreation therapists coach teenagers and young adults in dating, consent, expressing feelings, and how partnered sex works. And some behavior therapists talk with children, teenagers, and young adults about masturbation, making sure they understand how and where they can masturbate and places that are off-limits for masturbation, as well as how to clean up afterwards. If your child is over eighteen and on legal guardianship, their therapists may need your permission as a parent or guardian to provide specific information about sexual intimacy.

Q: What are the key messages I should share?
Although many aspects of sex education are similar for autistic kids and their neurotypical peers, autistic teens and young adults have pointed out areas ripe for improvement. Make sure to:

- **Prep them for puberty.** Knowing what to expect can help to reduce anxiety and give them a road map to understand the changes ahead. As their body begins to change, describe what the world around them may consider appropriate versus inappropriate conversation. I knew a woman whose daughter would regularly update her mom as to the pubertal changes she was experiencing. This resulted in frequent reports over breakfast along the lines of, "This morning I had two new pubic hairs!" The mom let her daughter know that while she was comfortable hearing that information, and shared her excitement in her bodily changes, such information would not be socially appropriate at school or with people she met in public (like grocery cashiers).

- **Go beyond reproduction.** Autistic teens and young adults often recall learning about the basic biology of reproduction but describe the social aspects of relationships and sexuality as having been neglected. Often, they want to learn about how to appropriately express dating or sexual interest in others, how to tell if someone is interested in them (or not), and how to manage sensory issues related to physical affection and intimacy. Offer books that cover social and relationship issues and not just biology basics.

- **Use specific terms.** As described in earlier chapters, I'm a big believer in making sure all children have language for their body parts. This is especially important when it comes to sexuality education for autistic people, who may be confused by the ways that neurodiverse people tend to talk around sex in vague, coded ways (e.g., *blow job, dirty talk, sleep together, giving head, home run, notches in their belt, body count, safer sex*). That said, do teach them the common meanings of slang terms (*ass, tits, blow job*, etc.) so that they understand what others are saying to or asking of them. This can help them feel more included and may also help them stay safer.

- **Discuss gender identity and sexual orientation.** Substantial percentages of autistic people identify as LGBTQ+. Make sure to approach these topics with love, openness, and curiosity rather than with shame, questions like "Are you sure?" or attempts to change their identity.

- **Avoid focusing on the problems.** Autistic adults are clear that, growing up, caregivers sometimes focused far too much on rare but serious risks such as running into legal problems for public masturbation, downloading child sexual abuse images, or stalking others. These are real issues that do need to be mentioned (as we do in this chapter); the key is not to make them the focus. Discussing those issues is more about legal education than sexuality education. When it comes to sexuality education, make sure to highlight sexual curiosity, pleasure, feelings, love, connection, intimacy, body exploration, and other good parts about sex too.

- **Describe why people have sex.** Autistic teens and young adults sometimes say that they spent a long time wondering why people have sex other than to become pregnant. Try to be direct about the fact that people have sex because it's fun, pleasurable, an expression of love, and/or helps people feel closer to one another. Similarly, people masturbate for many reasons, including because it's fun, feels good, or helps them to relax or fall asleep.

- **Normalize mistakes, rejection, and learning.** Sometimes people have very long gaps of time when they haven't asked anyone out or been romantic or sexual with another person. While it's perfectly fine to not be interested in dating or sex, some people are interested but had an incident that went sideways, and it made them too worried or scared to try again. Let your child know that everyone, with and without ASD, makes mistakes when it comes to sex and dating. It takes practice (and failure) to improve at anything, whether math, sports, kissing, or sex. Everyone gets their heart broken and experiences rejection sometimes. And far too many people (again, including neurotypical people) are laughed at or called a pervert when they share a sexual fantasy or desire with a friend or partner. It's also common to worry about having one's body judged or laughed at. I tell my students that if someone laughs at their body or ridicules their weight, penis size, breasts, pubic hair, vulva, thighs, or such, that behavior says nothing about their body, which is fine as it is. Rather, it means that the other person may still be learning that intimate partners could use kindness (or how to keep negative comments to themselves). "Their behavior is not about you," I emphasize. "It's about them and where they are in their learning." Further, condescending remarks may be relationship red flags; the person saying them may be trying to lower their partner's self-esteem to tip the balance of power in their favor, which is not okay.

- **Look for opportunities for socialization.** Making small talk, asking people to hang out, and sharing observations about the world (as well as personal feelings) are all good foundational skills for eventual dating. And these skills grow with practice. It can be easy to feel like one's child is happiest reading in their bedroom or hanging out on their computer, and while that may be true, in-person social opportunities (balanced with attention to potential sensory overload as well as a need for downtime) are valuable too. Best Buddies International, The Arc, and Special Olympics are options as are community activities focused on art, music, sports, or hobbies (crafting, knitting, chess).

- **Play to their strengths.** If your child is strong in understanding scientific concepts, it may be easy for them to understand some aspects of puberty, reproduction, how birth control methods work, or how STIs are passed or prevented. (In fact, they may find this fascinating.) If your teen or young adult takes comfort in rules and routines, then make sure that they know the "rules" for sex, such as how, if they are having intercourse, they should place a condom on the erect penis before it is inserted into the vagina or anus and that the condom should stay on until after ejaculation has occurred and the penis has been taken out of the vagina or anus. Provide enough detail, with specific terms, so that they understand it, step by step. If your child is a visual learner, check out condom demonstration diagrams online. Some people use social stories (a style of book commonly used to teach social skills) or comic book–style conversations to teach sex education. You can also practice with them using a penis model, which are sold online.

- **Avoid suggesting that relationships and sex will never be for them.** Many autistic individuals create pleasurable romantic and sexual lives whether they are living with family, friends, or in the community, and regardless of their use of verbal language. None of these circumstances determine a person's possibilities for dating, sex, love, or even marriage. Keep an open mind in terms of your child's desires for love, companionship, and intimacy.

Additionally, if your child is eighteen or over, be clear that they should not engage in any sexual behavior (whether online, through texting or apps, or in person) with someone who is under eighteen. Some autistic people form friendships with people who are younger than them due to developmental similarities. Friendship is one thing, but it's important to emphasize (repeatedly) that they should not talk in sexual ways with people under eighteen or have sex with people who are under eighteen. Also, tell your child or teen to alert you if an adult approaches them for sexual activity.

Q: I'm exhausted by my many roles as a parent, caregiver, and advocate. I am not sure I can take on the additional role of being their sex educator. What can I do?

Some parents aren't sure what to say when it comes to sex, and others are just exhausted and could use a little help, whether from friends or professionals. For parents who have the resources to hire a sexuality educator to teach their child about age- and developmentally appropriate relationship and sexuality education, the investment can be worth it. This can be done one-on-one. However, most people don't have the luxury of hiring personal consultants or educators to support this work. If you're connected to a local support group or social group, perhaps families can combine resources to hire a local sexuality educator. There are also inclusive sexuality education books and resources that groups might share or read through together.

Parents can also request that higher-level sex education be included in their child's Individual Education Program (IEP). IEPs have social/emotional goals, as well as transition planning. Your school's sex education curriculum should be delivered to and/or modified for your child. Or nudge your child's school to offer inclusive sexuality education as part of their larger educational plan. They may need to hire a sexuality educator or consultant who understands the sexuality education needs of autistic kids to deliver this more inclusive sex education and/or help the school revise and update their curriculum accordingly.

Sex therapists can also be helpful in supporting teens and young adults with anxiety around asking people out, assessing interest, and/or communicating sexual desires and needs. Health insurance covers sex therapy in certain circumstances, and some therapists offer sliding-scale fees. You can search for one in your area through the American Association of Sexuality Educators, Counselors and Therapists as well as the Society for Sex Therapy and Research (see **Resources**). Some providers offer virtual sessions, so there is a possibility of obtaining services even if you don't live in a city with a trained sex therapist. Recreational therapists can also be an important part of a caregiving team and may be covered by one's health insurance or state benefits program.

Q. What advice can you give me for a child with limited verbal skills? I don't even know what to talk about or how to present basic information. Every child is different. If you are not sure how to share information with your child, ask for advice from any professionals who may work with them. Some programs for autistic kids, such as the Autism Assessment, Research, Treatment, and Services (AARTS) Center at Rush Medical College in Chicago, have started to create visual sex education materials, and also lead relationship and sexuality education series for young teens, older teens, and young adults. If your community does not yet offer such services, perhaps families or local professionals (like recreational therapists and sex educators) can work together to expand available options.

SEXUALITY, SOCIAL SKILLS, AND ASKING PEOPLE OUT

Too often, autistic people are described as immature. This may contribute to misperceptions of autistic teens and adults as being uninterested in sex and/ or as having low sex drives. This can lead to autistic people feeling babied by others instead of treated as mature, sexy, and sexual people, many of whom are interested in romantic and sexual relationships, including the possibility of long-term partnering, marriage, and/or having children. That said, autistic individuals sometimes experience difficulties when it comes to expressing their romantic and/or sexual interest in others—more generally thought of as courtship. Some challenges involve what may be considered inappropriate courtship or "persistent courtship," which can feel worrisome or scary to the object of their affection.

In most instances, these courtship approaches are not meant to hurt, scare, or threaten the other person; rather, they often reflect the difficulty many autistic people experience in understanding what other people are thinking or feeling and/or detecting nonverbal cues that indicate someone isn't interested in them.[105] Courtship problems may also reflect differences in communication styles between autistic individuals and their non-autistic peers. For example, a non-autistic person might attempt to gently decline a request for a date by saying that they're "busy" or by saying "maybe some other night." While a non-autistic person might read between the lines and understand the person is not into them (if not after the first rejection, then at least by the second or third), an autistic person may not pick up on that cue and persist in asking their crush out, over and over again. Teach your child about how people communicate rejection. As painful as it is, they need to understand that when someone ghosts them, they should not continue trying to make contact. Also make sure your child knows that rejection is not a sign to give up on romantic and/or sexual relationships entirely (even if they do need to move on from a particular person), but to

learn, laugh, heal, and go forward. Rejection can feel especially disheart-
ening for people who have felt socially excluded, time and again—and can
be difficult not to take to heart—but nearly everyone gets over it with time.
Being overly cautious and hiding from the world is no way to learn and no
way to find a partner.

While persistent courtship may be perceived as stalking, another perspective might ask why more non-autistic people don't turn others down in
clearer ways. Sometimes there are good reasons for being vague. Women are
often socialized to let men down easily, as too many women are subjected
to verbal and physical aggression when they reject men. Also, some neurotypical people simply worry about hurting another's feelings. However,
autistic people often find it difficult to pick up on oblique language and
social norms. Talk with your child about the importance of communicating
directly when it comes to dating and sexual preferences.

Many autistic people have learned over time that social contact—whether
with classmates, friends, or coworkers—happens as a direct result of their
persistence. Because they may be less likely to be invited out with friends,
they may only get to hang out with people by following them or inviting
themselves along. One could argue whether this is adaptive or not; regardless, it's a truth of some people's lives. Accordingly, some autistic people
are more likely to express interest in a crush by following them or touching
them inappropriately. Studies show that significantly fewer autistic people
say they know how to initiate a relationship as compared to non-autistic
peers.[106] Again, better relationship and sexuality education could help.

Parents might tell their autistic child stories of times that they were
asked out or asked others out, including details such as how they could tell
that someone liked them, as well as how they may have tried to let someone
know they liked them or wanted to go on a date. If your child learns from
reading social stories, creating one for them or with them can be another
helpful approach. Such a story might include details like, "I can say, 'Would
you like to have lunch with me sometime?' If they say yes, I can ask for
their phone number and then text them to find a day that works for them.

If they don't respond to my text after two times, I should stop texting. Also, I should not contact them in other ways unless they call or text me first."

When it comes to text etiquette, it helps to have a guideline. Parents can say that if someone does not respond after two or three texts, their child shouldn't keep texting that person for a response. Otherwise, the person may feel bothered, harassed, or that they're being stalked. Parents can also support their child in teaching them how to recognize if someone is feeling bothered or harassed (they walk away, stop talking to them, don't respond to texts) and then suggest a rule that, if their child sees that happening, they should give that person space. They should also not approach or go to someone's home uninvited or follow them to class.

Non-autistic kids can use support and advice too. Sometimes people get in the habit of declining a date in polite but vague ways, even when they don't feel in danger. Anything they can say to be clear about their lack of interest, or to indicate that their "no" is final, may help. For example, saying "No thank you, I'm in a relationship" is clearer than "No thank you, I'm busy tonight," which may suggest they are interested but just not available that evening, and thus should be asked out again for tomorrow or next week. Saying "I appreciate you asking, but I am just not interested; please don't ask me again" can help make it clearer, too, especially if the person has asked once or twice before. Using nonspecific terms like "I'm just not feeling it" may be confusing.

If a person is feeling stalked, harassed, or threatened by a peer, they should seek help, whether from a parent, trusted adult, or—if they're in college—from the campus office that addresses stalking or harassment. At the same time, non-autistic students should learn that persistence does not always equate to being stalked, and that there might be an opportunity to stop behavior by using clear language. Saying "Please don't text me again" or "I don't like when you do this" are direct forms of communication that can be tried before considering next steps. Even though most autistic people mean no harm, they do sometimes need support in learning to respect boundaries.

⚖️ Mateo, a high-functioning autistic student at a prestigious university, wanted to spend time with Lilly, a friendly classmate. Lilly gave Mateo her phone number, and he began sending her texts with kittens and messages about strategies for online games. As time passed, Mateo developed a crush on Lilly and wanted to date her. Unfortunately for Mateo, Lilly had no interest in him as anything other than a casual friend. However, because she didn't want to hurt his feelings, whenever Mateo asked her to go to dinner or a movie with him, she just said she had plans or wasn't feeling well. Lilly did not clearly express to Mateo that she did not want to date him. When Mateo continued to invite her out and even began buying her small gifts, Lilly felt she had no option other than to ghost Mateo. Perplexed as to why Lilly stopped responding to his texts and why she wouldn't even say hi when she saw him on campus, Mateo persisted in texting, emailing, and direct messaging Lilly. He even began to wait for her outside of her classes and job. At that point, Lilly felt she had no choice other than to file a Title IX complaint against Mateo for stalking. Mateo's family hired Kristina and Susan to help navigate the complaint and help advocate for Mateo as a student with disabilities.

A surface review of the case would lead one to think that Mateo's behavior did, in fact, fit the definition of stalking and harassment. Though he never threatened Lilly (his messages were polite), the sheer volume of his communication and requests for her to go out with him were overwhelming. Kristina and Susan had to explain to Mateo in clear terms that by not responding to his texts or calls, what Lilly intended to communicate was that she did not want to be friends, much less have a romantic relationship. This explanation shocked Mateo, as he believed he had met a possible love match.

Kristina and Susan recognized that Mateo's actions towards Lilly were likely a reflection of having ASD rather than an unhealthy obsession with Lilly or a desire to cause Lilly to fear for her safety. Mateo was incredibly reluctant to reveal his ASD diagnosis to the Title IX investigator, but Kristina and Susan assured him that it was necessary to do so. Ultimately, Mateo and Lilly agreed to resolve the Title IX case through an informal resolution agreement that required Mateo to take social skills training classes. Mateo also had to agree to no longer attempt to communicate with Lilly in any fashion. Lilly felt relieved that she would no longer have to worry about being bombarded by messages from Mateo. She didn't want to see Mateo face discipline; she just wanted him to leave her alone.

SEXUAL PLEASURE, EXPLORATION, AND SENSORY ISSUES

Most autistic teens and young adults are interested in sexuality but all too often feel and are undereducated about sex, especially in the concrete ways they are most likely to understand. Depending on their age and developmental stage, as well as their sexual readiness, they may find it helpful to talk through potential rules for:

- **Admiring other people's bodies.** Some people (including those on the autism spectrum) have strong preferences for certain body parts—whether butts, breasts, chest, feet, arms, or any other part. Ask your child not to stare at people and also not to take pictures of others without first asking for and getting permission. Make sure your child knows that it is usually overstepping boundaries to take pictures of strangers' bodies even if you do ask first (such as going up to strangers and asking to take pictures of their breasts) as that may feel scary or harassing. Indeed, Kristina and Susan had a client on the spectrum who loved butts so much that he took pictures of his friends' butts without permission and was then devastated when those friends stopped socializing with him. He found it difficult to understand why an apology wouldn't return their friendships to normal and became depressed at the loss of those friendships. The women he photographed understood that their friend had ASD, and that the picture-taking was likely connected to that, but they just didn't want to continue having any contact with him, given the boundary he had crossed.

- **Respecting other people's bodies.** Because sexual touch and partnered sex can feel fun, pleasurable, and connecting, it may not be clear why people don't do it more often. Talk about respecting other people's boundaries, which includes not touching another person's body (and especially not their vulva, penis, butt, or breasts) without their permission.

- **Establishing boundaries for one's own body.** Thinking and talking through rules for one's own body may help people not be harmed or taken advantage of. Some autistic people describe feeling that others used them or tricked them, such as an acquaintance or someone they met at a party telling them that they were their boyfriend in order to get sex. Make sure they know that becoming a boyfriend or girlfriend takes time, such as several dates over weeks or months, and that such relationships should make them feel safe, good inside, and like they can be themselves. The reality is that autistic individuals are indeed at heightened risk of sexual victimization, which is not helped by a lack of inclusive sex education. As you would with any young person, make sure to have multiple conversations, time and again, about how to tell if someone is trying to trick a person or take advantage of them.

- **Openness and transparency.** With more autistic and non-autistic people alike exploring open relationships, polyamory, and consensual nonmonogamy, teens and young adults need to learn about the kinds of rules, communication, and transparency that these kinds of relationships—as well as monogamy—involve. Regardless of the relationship structure one chooses, partners should talk through what kinds of sex are okay to have with others (if any), how they will manage jealousy, safer sex strategies, and how they will communicate with one another (or not) about their sexual behaviors.

When it comes to making out and having sex, autistic teens and young adults can also be helped by specific information and tips to improve their experience. Thus, consider sharing these ideas (which most people can benefit from hearing, not just autistic people):

- Before kissing or making out, some people brush their teeth first, especially if they or their partner are sensitive to tastes and/or smells.

- Before getting naked together for partnered sex, some people shower first, especially if they or their partner are sensitive to smells or tastes or would just feel more comfortable clean.

- It's okay to avoid open-mouthed kissing or other forms of affection or sexual sharing if one or more partners doesn't like them.

- Using latex (or non-latex) gloves can be helpful if there's a sensation they don't like, such as vaginal wetness as part of fingering.

- Some people find it helpful to plan out or "schedule" sex so they can find a time when they and their partner are more likely to be relaxed or can set aside time to focus on one another.

- Many couples find it helpful to build downtime into their day, which can support their overall relationship as well as their sex life. For some people, this means taking time between work/school and going on dates to just be quiet and alone. For those who live together, it may mean spending time in different rooms before reconnecting with the other person for planned affection or sexual intimacy.

- People whose bodies are not very sensitive may find that using a multispeed vibrator helps to enhance sensation.

- People whose bodies are prone to sensory overload, including painful response to touch, may find it helpful to reduce sensation by keeping most of their clothes on, using blankets in between their bodies, or taking breaks from partnered touch every now and then.

- It's also okay to have quick sex if that's what both partners want. Sex is not always a long, drawn-out affair.

- Penile-vaginal intercourse isn't for everyone. Some people delay intercourse until they are in love or married. Some don't like the way it makes them worry about pregnancy risk, and others just don't like how vaginal intercourse feels for their body. Have the kinds of sex you like and don't worry about having the kinds you or your partner don't like.

- Adults who want to become pregnant but do not like the feeling of vaginal intercourse can do what many couples with vaginismus (a condition in which vaginal penetration feels painful if not impossible) do, which is ejaculate near the entrance to the vagina and then move the semen inside, or talk with a doctor about intrauterine insemination or other fertility procedures. Some people get creative by ejaculating into a condom or diaphragm and then inserting it into the vagina to get the sperm closer to the cervix.

Some autistic people find it helpful to communicate with their partner(s) in very specific ways. Yet, sexual communication looks different for different people. Some will use verbal language to share what they like and what they don't like, as well as the intensities and durations of the kinds of touch or sex they enjoy. Some write out their sex instructions or personal "tips" for their partner. Others use assisted communication devices, pictures, or diagrams to share their sexual likes and dislikes. Specific instructions help others learn what makes their partner feel good, bad, comfortable, in pain, or overstimulated.

A young woman with an autistic partner shared some of the ways she and her partner adjusted their sexual experiences to meet their sensory needs. "My partner doesn't like the feeling of hair on their mouth," she said, "so they're very against performing oral, because it causes them a lot of sensory issues. Also, sometimes certain, like, sounds . . . like, some of the wet noises that occur [during sex], it's just too much. And it doesn't tend to bother them as much when they're, when they're receiving it, 'cause they probably don't hear it as much as when they're closer to where it's all occurring, as would happen with giving oral." Additionally, she shared that her partner doesn't like the feeling of lubricant on their hands, so they use latex gloves. While these steps might seem like a lot, they show how people can adjust sex to their or their partner's comfort zone. Whether it's having sex with the lights dimmed (or completely off) or having sex only after taking a shower, brushing teeth, or grooming one's pubic hair, most people have preferred conditions for sex.

Finally, try to normalize that it's common for people to benefit from thoughtful and intentional approaches to their sex lives. Some people may feel like they have to go about their sex lives in ways they'd seen in movies or in pornography. This may mean insisting on intercourse, even if they're not really into it. Or feeling like sex should be wordless, even though in real life people may talk, laugh, get the hiccups, or tell a partner that something hurts and they need to stop. Share that sex looks lots of different ways and that it changes throughout life. People are always adjusting sex to suit their own or their partner's emotional and physical needs.

WHAT KINK HAS TO DO WITH IT

As we've described throughout this book, people have expectations when it comes to sex, and those are not always explicitly communicated. Yet, sex tends to be more fun, pleasurable, and clearly consensual when people talk openly, share what they like and dislike, ask their partner(s) what they like and dislike, and ask what kinds of sex are okay and not okay to do. Fortunately, many autistic individuals thrive on frank communication and have a desire to clearly understand rules. It can help to frame sexual communication in terms of rules and boundaries that are about safety as well as rules and boundaries that are about pleasure and joy.

Young autistic people have the same curiosities as any other young adult, so it comes as no surprise to many sexuality educators and therapists—though it does surprise some parents—when autistic teens and young adults spend time on kink or BDSM websites, message boards, or pornography, or otherwise express an interest in kink or fetish communities.* Colleagues who are sex therapists share that they are often contacted by parents who have learned their teen has been watching kink or fetish-oriented pornography or has been visiting related websites. Sometimes their teen happens to share with them that they've developed an interest in these kinds of sex, whether they use terms like BDSM, kink, or alt-sex, or describe being into fetishes, bondage, domination, submission, restraints, rope play, or such.

Given the harmful stereotypes about BDSM/kink in mainstream television and movies, learning that their teen or young adult has developed such interests worries some parents. Others are not so concerned, especially if they understand such interests are quite common and that anyone can be interested in sexual variety and kink (*Fifty Shades of Grey* was a worldwide phenomenon for good reasons). However, there's some evidence that autistic people may be more likely to develop an interest in learning about kink and BDSM for many reasons,[107] including that such communities tend to:

- Teach about the importance of open sexual communication and consent.
- Offer adults a chance to learn, whether through workshops or social gatherings, how to engage in kink play safely and consensually.
- Feel like safe spaces in which to explore gender roles and expressions.
- Value clear communication about limits and boundaries as well as respecting one another's limits and boundaries.
- Offer a sense of community, belonging, and identity.
- Accept and embrace people who are sexually interested in specific body parts (e.g., butts, feet, hands) or nonhuman objects (e.g., gloves, panties) or specific materials (e.g., lace, latex, leather), rather than making them feel weird or ashamed for their turn-ons.

---

* Please note: BDSM and kink communities are not the same as the mainstreaming of rough sex, which we described in Chapter 7 and which does not tend to be characterized by such careful communication, structure, rules, or opportunities for classes or workshops.

- Offer opportunities for sensory exploration. Some types of play (e.g., flogging, slapping) may be pleasurable for those who are hyposensitive or have high pain thresholds. Additionally, those who find pleasure, calm, or a sense of release from tight hugs might also enjoy being bound.

If your autistic teen or young adult seems to have developed an interest in diverse forms of sexual expression, don't panic and do express curiosity and openness to learning. In discovering kink or BDSM, they may have stumbled upon a form of sexual expression that offers structure, frank communication, acceptance, and opportunities to have their sensory needs met or at least understood.

PORNOGRAPHY, MASTURBATION, AND SEX

In addition to the information about pornography presented in Chapter 6, there are some special considerations when it comes to autistic kids watching pornography. Pornography is one of the nonsocial sources that young autistic people may turn to in order to learn about bodies, sex, and relationships. Additionally, some autistic kids may watch pornography somewhat often, especially if they find it challenging to connect with others offline. This makes it extra important to let them know that pornography is not real sex—that it features paid actors, pretend dialogue, and sex that tends to be more aggressive than in real life.

Depending on the kinds of sex your teen or young adult child is interested in, they may benefit from some additional specific information, such as that it's a good idea to use condoms for intercourse with new partners and that anal sex usually feels better with lots of lubricant (and more time to prepare, as well as going more slowly at first). If they have sensory issues that lead to them feeling overstimulated or in pain from too much touch, or from certain parts being touched, it may help them to learn that when people have sex, their bodies often touch in multiple places (faces, chests, legs) and not just where their genitals meet. Hearing that sex tends to look different in real life than it does in mainstream movies or pornography often helps too. For example, many young autistic adults find it a relief to hear that, in real life, people tend to take some time to put on a condom, that it can be easier to keep an erection if a partner applies the condom and then adds water-based lubricant to the condom-covered penis, and that people sometimes fart or burp during sex, or take breaks if they have a leg cramp or experience sensory overload.

Also, be specific about where and when it's okay to masturbate. A common refrain is to teach children to masturbate somewhere private, such as in a bedroom or bathroom. But some people need additional guidance to understand what privacy looks like in a college setting, where they may share a room with someone. During the Q&A part of a lecture at a conference geared toward parents and kids on the spectrum, a young adult once asked Kristina and Susan, "What's the problem with masturbating in your dorm room if it's okay to masturbate in your bedroom? Isn't my dorm room my bedroom?" They clarified that if it's a shared space with a roommate, then it's not the same as a single bedroom. Some people also teach that *private* means when you can't see anyone else, which can help to prevent situations like someone masturbating in their home but while standing at a window, or masturbating on a bus (where they might otherwise feel like it's private if they have the row to themselves).

The Internet and the Law

Kristina and Susan note that parents of autistic tweens and teens may want to occasionally monitor their social media use (as with neurotypical kids, in open and transparent ways). Although rare, some autistic students are adept at gaining access to the dark web, as well as other chat apps that would be difficult for most people to figure out how to access. Many are simply looking for friends and then find themselves watching pornography. However,

Kristina and Susan have represented many young adults who found themselves unknowingly involved in the unlawful solicitation of minors or raided by police for viewing child pornography. Some young people with low IQs may get aroused when engaging in sexual discussions and not realize they are speaking with minors. Other times they may realize someone is a minor, but not comprehend the potential harms related to sexual conversations with people who are underage. Sadly, some clients just wanted to talk to someone and don't really understand how their engagement in the dark web even happened.

In Kristina and Susan's professional experience, extra precautions are especially wise when young people remain online for hours upon hours, as lacking face-to-face socialization or opportunities to meet people who would be well suited for friendship or even a dating relationship can increase risk. Those who lack real, live friendships become especially vulnerable to online predators, who sometimes entice disabled students into conversations that would never have occurred in the context of a typical friendship. All that said, these are rare scenarios, and online forums and message boards also create meaningful and important social connections for many young people. With a few guardrails (filters, family rules, open communication, and mutual agreements for occasional technology spot checks), there can be far more upsides to technology use than downsides.

Collective Wisdom

Although not everyone wants to be romantic or sexual with other people, most people (including most autistic teens and young adults) are interested in these aspects of life. Here are some ways you can support your child on their journey:

1. **Autistic kids—like all kids—need sex education.** Although the burden is often placed on parents, school-based sex education should be more

inclusive, and educational plans are a place to address plans for such education. Sex educators, coaches, and therapists who have experience working with autistic people can help.

2. **It helps to talk early and often, and to be clear.** Start talking about puberty years before you expect it to happen to your child, as repetition may help them feel prepared. Also, avoid euphemisms and use clear language.

3. **Focus on the positives.** While it's important to know what kinds of things can go wrong, sex offers far more positives than negatives. Make sure to teach your child about pleasure, exploration, and the other emotional aspects of love, sexuality, and healthy relationships.

4. **Let your child know you believe in them.** If they want to go on dates or have a relationship, talk as if it's possible, because it often is. Follow this up by sharing information about healthy relationship characteristics, body boundaries, public versus private sexual behavior, STIs, and birth control, as well as how to tell when people are interested (or not interested). And of course, if your child is not interested in romantic relationships or sexuality, support them in that choice too.

CONCLUSION

Thank you for allowing me, Kristina, and Susan to be a part of your parenting journey. The choice to become a more askable and informed parent is a gift to your child. We acknowledge the magnitude of the information we've shared here, as well as the weight of some it. We've covered some difficult terrain at times. I hope that you will feel more prepared and more confident in your ability to support your child as they learn about their body, relationships, and sexuality. As you try on more conversations for size, here are a few closing thoughts:

First, respect where you are in the journey. Dr. Carol Dweck's concept of the "growth mindset" applies here, as it takes time to learn about sex and what it looks like for young people today, and it takes practice to have these talks with one's child. If you're feeling uncomfortable with these conversations, it may be because you're new to them. Or perhaps you're feeling the lingering effects of being raised in sexual silence or shame. You may be working to unlearn patterns at the same time as you work to acquire new skills, terminology, and ideas. That's a lot to do at once; self-care and compassion are important.

Second, take the long view. *Yes, Your Kid* is meant to support you and your family across multiple ages and stages. No one can cover everything at once; it would be overwhelming for both you and your child. You might find it helpful to come up with concrete steps. Try choosing one way to weave in more sexuality conversations and put it into practice. Will you start by talking about bodies and sex for five minutes a week? Giving your child an age-appropriate book about bodies or sexuality? Sitting down with your smartphone-owning teen to talk about pornography?

Third, consider your own guiding principles and values when navigating complex issues with your child. These might include leading with love and support, appreciating their curiosity about bodies and sexuality, trusting your child with factual information about their bodies or sexuality, or being nonjudgmental about your older teen's or young adult's sexual choices (which are likely to be different than yours in some way; it's a different time and they are their own person). Where possible, avoid doom-and-gloom language ("Having sex before marriage will ruin your life!" or "If you send someone a nude image, it will follow you around forever and destroy your reputation!"). Even though there are good reasons to give firm warnings about certain topics—and those warnings vary from family to family, influenced by religious and cultural belief systems—this can be done in a way that is informative and not fear-based. One concern about fear tactics (aside from the fact that they rarely work) is that young people will feel unable to turn to their parents should something go wrong. What children of all ages need more than anything is unconditional love from their parents—to know that they have someone who will listen to them, celebrate their wins, and help them navigate difficulties (and especially crises). I often think of a friend whose family adopted the motto "We can do hard things together," and the ways they use it as a touchstone to return to when life feels its hardest.

Fourth, try not to go it alone. Jessica Grose, *New York Times* columnist and author of *Screaming on the Inside*, has noted how much work parents—and especially mothers, in families that include one—tend to shoulder. In addition to packing lunches, driving carpools, planning birthday parties, and managing doctors' appointments for our children, parents are often their child's primary sex educators. Yet, as Byllye Avery has highlighted through her work with the Black Women's Health Imperative, collective problems require collective solutions. Parents need the support of their communities. Comprehensive school-based sexuality education is needed because it's important not just for my child and your child to be informed about sex, birth control, STI testing and treatment, healthy relationships, mutual pleasure, and consent, but for all of the teens and young adults in one's community to have age-appropriate sexuality education and foundational knowledge. Where school-based sexuality education is not possible, consider banding together with other parents to nudge community youth organizations to incorporate thoughtful sexuality education into their curricula. Consider hosting a speaker series on the topics we have discussed or start a parent-teen conversation circle, where you take turns hosting and rotate topics that your group of families feels are important to discuss.

Finally, I want to leave you with some quotes from college students from across the US responding to a question I posed about how parents can better support their teens when it comes to sexuality issues. After all, they're closer to adolescence than I've been in some time, and I value their expertise. They wrote:

"Children need to know that their parents have their back and will help them with any questions or concerns. If parents are not okay with talking to their children about sex then the children are more apt to sneak around and potentially end up getting pregnant or an STD. It might be an awkward conversation at first, but once you break the ice, children will feel more comfortable talking to [you] or asking questions. I know I was."

"Abstinence-only education does not work. Teach me how to set boundaries and not feel shame in having sexual pleasure."

"Students need to be educated on what a healthy relationship looks like, because those are the sort of relationships that are rarely shown in the media."

"Be willing to buy condoms and birth control, and not make their child feel embarrassed about sex."

"Parents need to be more open to the fact that their kid is going to eventually have sex. A lot of times, sex makes parents uncomfortable because they don't want to imagine their kid ever doing that, but in reality it's natural and they need to get over the tension and have conversations so that their kids know what's ok to do and what's not. Sexual thoughts and behaviors naturally occur throughout childhood and not knowing how to respond to those feelings can be confusing if no one has ever said anything about it before."

"I think parents know that we are having sex so maybe just let the parents be more open about it and talk to their children more. You really can't do anything to prevent sex since mostly everyone is sexually active. So, if parents would sit down and talk with their kids about how they can be safer, that might help."

My experiences working with young people have shown me how excited and joyful they often feel about exploring relationships, intimacy, and sexuality. There's nothing quite like those first few flirtations and crushes, learning another person's heart, or figuring out affection and intimacy with someone who's also new to it all. Awkward? Yes. But those are also the days about which countless songs and poems have been written, and they can be a wonder to witness. Young people have plenty of concerns and anxieties, too, which can often be eased when they have a parent or caregiver they can turn to for love, support, and accurate information.

You may or may not talk with your child about each of the topics in this book, and that's okay. And, even if you do, your child may not always listen to you—but at least they will hear your voice and know that you are trying. With every conversation, you have a chance to show your child that you love them, and you want so many good things for them in life that you're willing to take on some awkward moments in exchange for offering them information, guidance, and support. In front of you, there's a journey of a hundred conversations—many brief, others more involved—as you give your child more tools to help them create a life that feels good to them. This is just the beginning.

RESOURCES

FIND A PROFESSIONAL

American Association of Sexuality Educators, Counselors, and Therapists (AASECT)

Includes a directory to find AASECT-certified sexuality educators, counselors, and therapists who are working in the US and internationally.

AASECT.org

Elevatus Training

Offers trainings for parents, schools, and professionals related to sexuality, disabilities, and autism.

ElevatusTraining.com

Society for Sex Therapy and Research

Includes a directory to find sex therapists in one's local area.

SSTARnet.org

Women of Color Sexual Health Network

Features a directory to identify sexuality professionals in various geographic areas.

WoCSHN.org

EDUCATIONAL RESOURCES FOR FAMILIES

Amaze

Videos for parents, tweens, and teens about puberty, relationships, and sexuality topics.

Amaze.org

American Sexual Health Association

Resources on diverse sexual health and relationship topics.

ASHASexualHealth.org

Autism Assessment, Research, Treatment, and Services (AARTS)

Resources, educational programs, and clinic care for young people with autism.

Rush.edu/services/autism-care

Birds + Bees + Kids

Sex education resources for families.

BirdsandBeesandKids.com/sex-education-resources-parents-kids/

Centers for Disease Control and Prevention

Includes STD fact sheets and brochures.

CDC.gov

Children and Screens: Institute of Digital Media and Child Development

Offers a parent-focused "Ask the Experts" webinar series that can be viewed online.

ChildrenandScreens.com

Common Sense Media

Includes television and movie reviews as well as information on parental controls and filters/settings to restrict online content.

CommonSenseMedia.org

Culture Reframed Parents Program

Resources for parents to support conversations about pornography, healthy relationships, and technology use.

Parents.CultureReframed.org

In the Know

Free downloadable materials for teens and young adults that address topics such as sexting, pornography, choking, rough sex, mental health, and body image.

InTheKnow.co.nz

It Gets Better Project

Includes a Queer Sex Ed series of videos that center young LGBTQ+ people as well as videos created by LGBTQ+ adults describing their journeys of coming out and creating positive lives for themselves.

ItGetsBetter.org

It's Time We Talked

Australia-based organization featuring resources for parents, educators, and schools to engage with youth around pornography and other sexually explicit materials.

ItsTimeWeTalked.com

Love Is Respect

Youth-focused website that addresses healthy relationships, dating, safety, and provides information and resources related to dating violence and abuse.

LoveIsRespect.org

Making Caring Common Project

Includes free resources for parents on topics such as helping young people grow their empathy, learn from their mistakes, and combat sexual harassment.

MCC.gse.harvard.edu

Media Aware Parent

A sex and media literacy program for families.

MediaAwareParent.com

National Association for Media Literacy Education

Includes resources for parents to engage kids of all ages in asking questions about the media they create and consume.

NAMLE.net

National Sex Education Standards, Second Edition

Sexuality education standards, developed by professionals, along with suggestions for ages/grades for which such information may be most relevant.

AdvocatesforYouth.org/resources/health-information/future-of-sex
-education-national-sexuality-education-standards/

OutCare

Features a directory of LGBTQ+ affirming healthcare providers.

OutCareHealth.org

Parents and Caregivers as Sexuality Educators

A free downloadable curriculum offered by the Unitarian Universalist Association.

UUA.org/families/sexuality-educators

PFLAG

Information, educational resources, and support for families of LGBTQ+ individuals.

PFLAG.org

Planned Parenthood

Features fact sheets about birth control, reproductive health, and abortion.

PlannedParenthood.org

Safety Net Project

Provides resources, information, and support related to how technology can be used in the context of stalking, sexual assault, and intimate partner violence.

TechSafety.org

Sex, Etc.

A "by teens, for teens" sex education website.

SexEtc.org

Sex Positive Families

Education and podcasts to support families in raising sexually healthy children.

SexPositiveFamilies.com

Sexuality and Relationship Education for Families with Autistic Children

Resources on puberty and relationships from the National Autistic Society of the United Kingdom.

Autism.org.uk/advice-and-guidance/topics/family-life-and-relationships /sex-education/parents-and-carers

Stop It Now!

Provides support, information, and resources to keep children safe by preventing child sexual abuse.

StopItNow.org

Wait Until 8th

Provides information about a pledge for parents to delay giving their child a smartphone until at least eighth grade.

WaitUntil8th.org

What's OK?

Free, confidential resources (text, chat, phone, or email to connect with professional counselors) to help people who have concerns about sexual safety, boundaries, harm, or abuse.

WhatsOK.org

SUPPORT AND ADVOCACY

Advocates for Youth

Health information and resources for youth and their families, with a global reach.

AdvocatesforYouth.org

Gay, Lesbian, Bisexual, and Transgender National Hotline

Confidential access to resources and support.

1-888-843-4564

SIECUS: Sex Ed for Social Change

Features policy-related information related to sexuality education.

SIECUS.org

The Trevor Project

Offers information, support, and crisis services for young LGBTQ+ people.

TheTrevorProject.org

BOOKS

Preschool Through Early Elementary

All Bodies Are Good Bodies: A Children's Book About Body Positivity, Margaret Lynn Samora

Amazing You! Getting Smart About Your Private Parts, Gail Saltz and Lynne Cravath

C Is for Consent, Eleanor Morrison and Faye Orlove

Consent (for Kids!): Boundaries, Respect, and Being in Charge of YOU! Rachel Brian

Don't Touch My Hair, Sharee Miller

It's So Amazing! A Book About Eggs, Sperm, Birth, Babies and Families, Robie Harris and Michael Emberley

My Body! What I Say Goes! Jayneen Sanders and Farimah Khavarinezhad

Super Duper Safety School: Safety Rules for Kids & Grown-Ups, Pattie Fitzgerald

These Are My Eyes, This Is My Nose, This Is My Vulva, These Are My Toes, Lexx Brown-James

What Makes a Baby Cory Silverberg and Fiona Smyth

Yes! No! A First Conversation about Consent, Megan Madison, Jessica Ralli, and Isabel Roxas

For Puberty and Early Adolescence

The Autism-Friendly Guide to Periods, Robyn Steward

Body Drama: Real Girls, Real Bodies, Real Issues, Real Answers, Nancy Amanda Redd

Celebrate Your Body (And Its Changes Too!): The Ultimate Puberty Book for Girls, Sonya Renee Taylor

Growing Up Great! The Ultimate Puberty Book for Boys, Scott Todnem

Let's Talk About Sex: Changing Bodies, Growing Up, Sex, Gender and Sexual Health (20th anniversary edition), Robie Harris and Michael Emberley

Puberty Is Gross but Also Really Awesome, Gina Loveless and Lauri Johnston

Sex Is a Funny Word: A Book About Bodies, Feelings, and You Cory Silverberg and Fiona Smyth

Vagina and Periods 101: A Pop-Up Book, Christian Hoeger and Kristen Lilla (at sexedtalk.com/product/vaginas-and-periods-101-a-pop-up-book/)

Wait, What? A Comic Book Guide to Relationships, Bodies, and Growing Up, Heather Corinna, Isabella Rotman, and Luke Howard

You-ology: A Puberty Guide for Every Body, Melisa Holmes, Trish Hutchison, and Kathryn Lowe

For Teenagers

Let's Talk About It: The Teen's Guide to Sex, Relationships, and Being a Human, Erika Moen and Matthew Nolan

You Know, Sex: Bodies, Gender, Puberty and Other Things, Cory Silverberg and Fiona Smyth

For Young Adults

The Book of Happy, Positive, and Confident Sex for Adults on the Autism Spectrum and Beyond! Michael John Carley and Ha! (at neurodiversitypress.com)

Drawn to Sex Volume 1: The Basics, Erika Moen and Matthew Nolan

Drawn to Sex Volume 2: Our Bodies and Health, Erika Moen and Matthew Nolan

For Parents

Behind Their Screens: What Teens Are Facing (and Adults Are Missing), Emily Weinstein and Carrie James

Boys & Sex: Young Men on Hookups, Love, Porn, Consent, and Navigating the New Masculinity, Peggy Orenstein

The Emotional Lives of Teenagers: Raising Connected, Capable, and Compassionate Adolescents, Lisa Damour

For Goodness Sex: Changing the Way We Talk to Teens about Sexuality, Values, and Health, Al Vernacchio

Girls & Sex: Navigating the Complicated New Landscape, Peggy Orenstein

Good Inside: A Guide to Becoming the Parent You Want to Be, Becky Kennedy

How to Raise Kids Who Aren't Assholes: Science-Based Strategies for Better Parenting—From Tots to Teens, Melinda Wenner Moyer

iGen: Why Today's Super Connected Kids Are Growing Up Less Rebellious, More Tolerant, Less Happy—and Completely Unprepared for Adulthood, Jean Twenge

Sex Positive Talks to Have with Kids: A Guide to Raising Sexually Healthy, Informed, Empowered Young People, Melissa Pintor Carnagey

Shameless Parenting: Everything You Need to Raise Shame-Free, Confident Kids and Heal Your Shame Too, Tina Schermer Sellers

The Talk: Helping Your Kids Navigate Sex in the Real World, Alice Dreger

To Raise a Boy: Classrooms, Locker Rooms, Bedrooms, and the Hidden Struggles of American Boyhood, Emma Brown

Under Pressure: Confronting the Epidemic of Stress and Anxiety in Girls, Lisa Damour

Untangled: Guiding Teenage Girls Through the Seven Transitions into Adulthood, Lisa Damour

ACKNOWLEDGMENTS

From Debby:

I'm grateful to my agent, Kari Stuart, for believing in this book from the beginning and for her thoughtful feedback on multiple rounds of proposals. Thanks, too, to Cat Shook and Phoebe Rhinehart for their support. The entire BenBella team has been outstanding to work with. I am grateful to my editor Leah Wilson, whose clear communication, insightful questions, and kind spirit have made writing this book a joy. Huge thanks, too, to Sarah Avinger and her team for their work on the cover design; to Jennifer Canzeroni and Alicia Kania for helping *Yes, Your Kid* makes its way into the world; to Kim Broderick for her design expertise; and to Scott Calamar for his careful copy editing.

To the thousands of teenagers and young adults who took part in my research studies: I am forever grateful to you for helping me better understand your world. I hope this book supports you and your families in creating helpful conversations. To the many parents who have shared with me funny anecdotes and big and small questions, as well as joyful and even painful experiences: Thank you for trusting me with your family's stories. And to the teachers, counselors, and therapists who help children understand their bodies, learn about consent, build resilience in the face of rejection, and create healthy friendships and relationships: Your work is vital.

I am fortunate to be surrounded by colleagues and students who have encouraged or collaborated with me on research, helped me make sense of our findings, and/or inspired me with their own work: Heather Eastman-Mueller, Tsung-chieh Fu, Lucia Guerra-Reyes, Jen Piatt, Paul Wright, Samantha Keene, Emily Rothman, Kim Nelson, Megan Maas, Dennis Fortenberry, Dubravka Svetina Valdivia, Cristina Ljungberg, Wendy Anderson, Catherine Sherwood-Laughlin, Eric Walsh-Buhi, Callie Patterson, Keisuke Kawata, Molly Rosenberg, John Feiner, Dan Savage, Peggy Orenstein, Jill Bauer, Ronna Gradus, Mary Balle, Dasha Carver, Owen Miller, Joan Tabachnick, Jonathon Beckmeyer, Marie Crabbe, Nikki Denholm, Nicola Gavey, Melanie Beres, Michael Seto, Kristen Jozkowski, Kate Julian, Bryant Paul, Zoë Peterson, Yael Rosenstock Gonzalez, Evan Theis, Sally Thomas, Sari van Anders, Eva Voorheis, Jodi Wilson, Brittanni Wright, Leila Wood, Devon Hensel, Shahzarin Khan, Ruhun Wasata, and Nelson Zounlome. My apologies for any omissions; there have been so many wonderful people who have been a part of this journey. Also, I'm grateful to Dean David Allison for pulling together a phenomenal crew of sexual health researchers at the IU School of Public Health-Bloomington.

My friends and family have been a lifeline, both during the COVID-19 pandemic and while writing this book; some even served as early readers despite their busy schedules. Huge thanks to Anna, Brittany, Catherine, Elaine, Jen, Laura, and Mary: Your support and solidarity mean the world to me. Finally, all my love and gratitude to my family of origin as well as my husband and our children. Every day, I am thankful for you and love you even more.

From Kristina and Susan:

A special thank you to our colleagues at Kohrman Jackson & Krantz, and to Jon Pinney, our managing partner, who has supported this project from day one. Susan would like to thank her friends, Wendy, Bridgette and Shari, who served as "readers" and put their whole hearts into providing us with feedback. To Sindy, thank you for always celebrating our achievements.

Kristina would like to thank Matt, and Susan would like to thank David, our spouses, each of whom has supported us through this venture as work on this book took place during evenings and weekends. Kristina would like her children to know they can always talk to her about whatever issues arise in life. Susan would like to thank her son-in-law and her step-daughter for entering her fold, and her original three children for giving her the opportunity to be that "askable" parent and for bringing meaning to each day.

ENDNOTES

1. Herbenick, D., Fu, T. C., and Hensel, D. Unpublished data from the 2018 National Survey of Sexual Health and Behavior.
2. Widman, L., Choukas-Bradley, S., Noar, S. M., Nesi, J., and Garrett, K. (2016). "Parent-adolescent sexual communication and adolescent safer sex behavior: A meta-analysis." *JAMA Pediatrics 170*(1): 52–61.
3. Alt, D., and Boniel-Nissim, M. (2018). "Parent-adolescent communication and problematic internet use: The mediating role of fear of missing out (FoMO)." *Journal of Family Issues 39*(13): 3391–3409; De Looze, M., Constantine, N. A., Jerman, P., Vermeulen-Smit, E., and ter Bogt, T. (2015). "Parent-adolescent sexual communication and its association with adolescent sexual behaviors: A nationally representative analysis in the Netherlands." *Journal of Sex Research 52*(3): 257–268.
4. 2019 Youth Risk Behavior Survey.
5. 2022 National Survey of Sexual Health and Behavior.
6. Higgins, J. A., Trussell, J., Moore, N. B., and Davidson Sr., K. J. (2010). "The language of love?—Verbal versus implied consent at first heterosexual intercourse: Implications for contraceptive use." *American Journal of Health Education 41*(4): 218–230.
7. Warshowsky, H., Mosley, D. V., Mahar, E. A., and Mintz, L. (2020). "Effectiveness of undergraduate human sexuality courses in enhancing women's sexual functioning." *Sex Education 20*(1): 1–16; Henry, D. S. (2013). "Couple reports of the perceived influences of a college human

sexuality course: an exploratory study." *Sex Education 13*(5): 509–521; Rogers, A., McRee, N., and Arntz, D. L. (2009). "Using a college human sexuality course to combat homophobia" *Sex Education 9*(3): 211–225; Fischer, G. J. (1986). "College student attitudes toward forcible date rape: Changes after taking a human sexuality course." *Journal of Sex Education and Therapy 12*(1): 42–46.

8. Weis, D. L., Rabinowitz, B., and Ruckstuhl, M. F. (1992). "Individual changes in sexual attitudes and behavior within college-level human sexuality courses." *Journal of Sex Research 29*(1): 43–59.

9. Martino, S. C., Elliott, M. N., Corona, R., Kanouse, D. E., and Schuster, M. A. (2008). "Beyond the 'big talk': The roles of breadth and repetition in parent-adolescent communication about sexual topics." *Pediatrics 121*(3): e612–e618.

10. SIECUS (2018). "On Our Side: Public Support for Sex Education." Retrieved from: https://siecus.org/wp-content/uploads/2018/08/On-Our-Side-Public-Support-for-Sex-Ed-2018-Final.pdf.

11. Evans, R., Widman, L., Kamke, K., and Stewart, J. L. (2020). "Gender differences in parents' communication with their adolescent children about sexual risk and sex-positive topics." *Journal of Sex Research 57*(2): 177–188.

12. Elliot, M., Browne, K., and Kilcoyne, J. (1995). "Child sexual abuse prevention: What offenders tell us." *Child Abuse & Neglect 19*(5): 574–594.

13. Burrows, K. S., Bearman, M., Dion, J., and Powell, M. B. (2017). "Children's use of sexual body part terms in witness interviews about sexual abuse." *Child Abuse & Neglect 65*: 226–235.

14. Gay, R. (2022). "The Struggle to Say No." The Audacity. Retrieved from: https://audacity.substack.com/p/the-struggle-to-say-no

15. Strachan, E., and Staples, B. (2012). "Masturbation." *Pediatrics in Review 33*(4): 190–191.

16. Armstrong, E. A., England, P., and Fogarty, A. C. (2012). "Accounting for women's orgasm and sexual enjoyment in college hookups and relationships." *American Sociological Review 77*(3): 435-462.

17. Chadwick, S. B., Francisco, M., and van Anders, S. M. (2019). "When orgasms do not equal pleasure: Accounts of "bad" orgasm experiences

during consensual sexual encounters." *Archives of Sexual Behavior 48*: 2435-2459.

18. Levin, R. J., and van Berlo, W. (2004). "Sexual arousal and orgasm in subjects who experience forced or non-consensual sexual stimulation—a review." *Journal of Clinical Forensic Medicine 11*(2): 82–88.

19. Lindberg, L. D., Firestein, L., and Beavin, C. (2021). "Trends in US adolescent sexual behavior and contraceptive use, 2006-2019." *Contraception: X 3*: 100064.

20. McCarthy, J. (2022). "Same-sex marriage support inches up to new high of 71 percent." Retrieved from: https://news.gallup.com/poll/393197 /same-sex-marriage-support-inches-new-high.aspx.

21. American Library Association (2022). "Large majorities of voters oppose book bans and have confidence in libraries." Retrieved from: https://www .ala.org/news/press-releases/2022/03/large-majorities-voters-oppose -book-bans-and-have-confidence-libraries.

22. Batteiger, T. A., Jordan, S. J., Toh, E., Fortenberry, L., Williams, J. A., LaPradd, M., Katz, B., Fortenberry, J. D., Dodge, B., Arno, J., Batteiger, B. E., and Nelson, D. E. (2019). "Detection of rectal Chlamydia trachomatis in heterosexual men who report cunnilingus." *Sexually Transmitted Diseases 46*(7): 440.

23. Basile, K. C., Clayton, H. B., DeGue, S., Gilford, J. W., Vagi, K. J., Suarez, N. A., Zwald, M. L., and Lowry, R. (2020). "Interpersonal violence victimization among high school students—Youth Risk Behavior Survey, United States, 2019." *MMWR supplements 69*(1): 28.

24. Dukers, N. H., Bruisten, S. M., Van den Hoek, J. A. R., De Wit, J. B., Van Doornum, G. J., and Coutinho, R. A. (2000). "Strong decline in herpes simplex virus antibodies over time among young homosexual men is associated with changing sexual behavior." *American Journal of Epidemiology 152*(7): 666–673.

25. "HIV Treatment as Prevention" (2022). Division of HIV Prevention. Centers for Disease Control and Prevention. Retrieved from: https:// www.cdc.gov/hiv/risk/art/index.html.

26. Armstrong, N. R., and Wilson, J. D. (2006). "Did the 'Brazilian' kill the pubic louse?" *Sexually Transmitted Infections 82*(3): 265–266; Dholakia,

S., Buckler, J., Jeans, J. P., Pillai, A., Eagles, N., and Dholakia, S. (2014). "Pubic lice: an endangered species?" *Sexually Transmitted Diseases 41*(6): 388–391.

27. Torrone, E. A., Lewis, F. M., Kirkcaldy, R. D., Bernstein, K. T., Ryerson, A. B., de Voux, A., Oliver, S. E., Quilter, L. A., and Weinstock, H. S. (2021). "Genital mycoplasma, Shigellosis, Zika, Pubic Lice, and other sexually transmitted infections: Neither gone nor forgotten." *Sexually Transmitted Diseases 48*(4): 310–314.

28. American College of Obstetricians and Gynecologists (2020). "Your First Gynecologic Visit." Retrieved from: https://www.acog.org/womens -health/faqs/your-first-gynecologic-visit.

29. Power to Decide (formerly The National Campaign to Prevent Teen and Unplanned Pregnancy) (2015). "Survey Says: Hide the Birth Control."

30. "Contraceptive Options and Effectiveness—Most or Moderately Effective Contraception." Office of Population Affairs. Retrieved on March 1, 2023 from: https://opa.hhs.gov/contraceptive-options-and-effectiveness -highlight1-text-only.

31. Rubinsky, V., and Cooke-Jackson, A. (2017). "'Tell me something other than to use a condom and sex is scary': Memorable messages women and gender minorities wish for and recall about sexual health." *Women's Studies in Communication 40*(4): 379–400; Rubinsky, V., and Cooke-Jackson, A. (2021). "'It would be nice to know I'm allowed to exist': Designing ideal familial adolescent messages for LGBTQ women's sexual health." *American Journal of Sexuality Education 16*(2): 221–237.

32. Herbenick, D., Patterson, C., Lumsdaine, B., Fu, T. C., Williams, A., Ovide, T., Miller, O., Thomas, S., and Eastman-Mueller, H. (Under review). "'I just really didn't know what I was walking into': Scary sexual experiences in a campus-representative survey of undergraduate students."

33. Willis, M., Hunt, M., Wodika, A., Rhodes, D. L., Goodman, J., and Jozkowski, K. N. (2019). "Explicit verbal sexual consent communication: Effects of gender, relationship status, and type of sexual behavior." *International Journal of Sexual Health 31*(1): 60–70.

34. Herbenick, D., Fu, T. C., Arter, J., Sanders, S. A., and Dodge, B. (2018). "Women's experiences with genital touching, sexual pleasure, and orgasm: results from a US probability sample of women ages 18 to 94." *Journal of Sex & Marital Therapy 44*(2): 201–212.

35. "Why It's So Difficult to Leave." Retrieved on March 1, 2023 from: https://www.womenagainstabuse.org/education-resources/learn-about -abuse/why-its-so-difficult-to-leave.

36. Streng, T. K., and Kamimura, A. (2015). "Sexual assault prevention and reporting on college campuses in the US: A review of policies and recommendations." *Journal of Education and Practice 6*(3): 65–71.

37. Herbenick, D., Fu, T. C., Dodge, B., and Fortenberry, J. D. (2019). "The alcohol contexts of consent, wanted sex, sexual pleasure, and sexual assault: Results from a probability survey of undergraduate students." *Journal of American College Health 67*(2): 144–152.

38. Anderson, M., and Jiang, J. (2022). "Teens, social media & technology 2022." Pew Research Center. Retrieved from: https://www.pewresearch .org/internet/2022/08/10/teens-social-media-and-technology-2022/; Robb, M. (2019). "Tweens, teens, and phones: What our 2019 research reveals." Common Sense Media. Retrieved from: https://www.common sensemedia.org/kids-action/articles/tweens-teens-and-phones-what -our-2019-research-reveals.

39. Lardieri, A. (February 2018). "Teens are sexting more than ever." *US News & World Report*. Retrieved from: https://www.usnews.com/news /national-news/articles/2018-02-27/teens-are-sexting-more-than-ever; Strasburger, V. C., Zimmerman, H., Temple, J. R., and Madigan, S. (2019). "Teenagers, sexting, and the law." *Pediatrics 143*(5): e20183183.

40. Seto, M. C., Roche, K., Stroebel, M., Gonzalez-Pons, K., and Goharian, A. (2023). "Sending, receiving, and nonconsensually sharing nude or near-nude images by youth." *Journal of Adolescence 1*(14).

41. Clancy, E. M., Klettke, B., and Hallford, D. J. (2019). "The dark side of sexting—Factors predicting the dissemination of sexts." *Computers in Human Behavior 92*: 266–272.

42. *Child Sexual Abuse Material (CSAM)*. National Center for Missing & Exploited Children. Retrieved on February 15, 2023 from: https://www.missingkids.org/theissues/csam.

43. Jenco, M. (2019). "Researchers call for decriminalization of consensual teen sexting." *AAP News*. American Academy of Pediatrics. Retrieved from: https://publications.aap.org/aapnews/news/13369; Strasburger, V. C., Zimmerman, H., Temple, J. R., and Madigan, S. (2019). "Teenagers, sexting, and the law." *Pediatrics 143*(5).

44. Ojeda, M., and Del Rey, R. (2021). "Lines of action for sexting prevention and intervention: A systematic review." *Archives of Sexual Behavior 51*(3): 1–29.

45. Murray, P., Ashcraft, A., Berta, A. M., Chang, J., Coyle, K., Lanyon, M., Potter, S., and Downs, J. (2021). "Female adolescents who identify as bisexual or other sexuality categories engage in more sexting compared to both heterosexual and lesbian female peers." *Journal of Pediatric and Adolescent Gynecology 34*(2): 268.

46. Strohmaier, H., Murphy, M., and DeMatteo, D. (2014). "Youth sexting: Prevalence rates, driving motivations, and the deterrent effect of legal consequences." *Sexuality Research and Social Policy 11*(3): 245–255.

47. Strohmaier, Murphy, and DeMatteo, "Youth sexting."

48. Ojeda and Del Rey. "Lines of action for sexting prevention and intervention"

49. Thorburn, B., Gavey, N., Single, G., Wech, A., Calder-Dawe, O., and Benton-Greig, P. (March 2021). "To send or not to send nudes: New Zealand girls critically discuss the contradictory gendered pressures of teenage sexting." *Women's Studies International Forum 85*: 102448. Pergamon.

50. Johnsen, C. A. (March 2018). "Teen sexting—help for parents." AP News. Retrieved from: https://apnews.com/article/cee6bf6a64fa449a8be6438ea1dd20bc.

51. DeKeseredy, W. S. (2021). "Image-based sexual abuse: Social and legal implications." *Current Addiction Reports 8*(2): 330–335.

52. Maas, M. K., Cary, K. M., Clancy, E. M., Klettke, B., McCauley, H. L., and Temple, J. R. (2021). "Slutpage use among US college students:

the secret and social platforms of image-based sexual abuse." *Archives of Sexual Behavior 50*(5): 2203–2214.

53. Garrity, M., and Blinder, A. (March 2015). "Penn State University's Secret Facebook Photos May Lead to Criminal Charges." *New York Times*. Retrieved from: https://www.nytimes.com/2015/03/18/us/penn -state-fraternitys-secret-facebook-photos-may-lead-to-criminal-charges .html.

54. Weissbourd, R., Ross Anderson, T., Cashin, A., and McIntyre, J. "The Talk." Making Caring Common Project. Retrieved on July 13, 2022 from: https://static1.squarespace.com/static/5b7c56e255b02c683659fe43 /t/5bd51a0324a69425bd079b59/1540692500558/mcc_the_talk_final .pdf.

55. "#MeToo in Middle School." Retrieved on July 13, 2022 from: https:// www.amightygirl.com/blog?p=28874.

56. Weissbourd, R., et al. "The Talk."

57. Hill, C., and Kearl, H. "Crossing the line: Sexual harassment at school." American Association of University Women. Retrieved on July 13, 2022 from: https://www.aauw.org/resources/research/crossing-the-line-sexual -harassment-at-school/.

58. "6 Tips for Reducing and Preventing Misogyny and Sexual Harassment Among Teens and Young Adults" (2018). Making Caring Common Project. Retrieved from: https://mcc.gse.harvard.edu/resources-for-families /6-tips-parents-reducing-preventing-misogyny-sexual-harassment.

59. Vogels, E. A. (2020). "10 Facts about Americans and Online Dating." Pew Research Center. Retrieved from: https://www.pewresearch.org /fact-tank/2020/02/06/10-facts-about-americans-and-online-dating/.

60. Karasavva, V., and Noorbhai, A. (2021). "The real threat of deepfake pornography: A review of Canadian policy." *Cyberpsychology, Behavior, and Social Networking 24*(3): 203–209.

61. Gieseke, A. P. (2020). "The New Weapon of Choice: Law's Current Inability to Properly Address Deepfake Pornography." *Vanderbilt Law Review 73*: 1479; Harris, D. (2018). "Deepfakes: False pornography is here and the law cannot protect you." *Duke Law & Technology Review 17*: 99.

62. Lee, S., Lohrmann, D. K., Luo, J., and Chow, A. (2022). "Frequent social media use and its prospective association with mental health problems in a representative panel sample of US adolescents." *Journal of Adolescent Health* 70(5): 796–803.
Social Media and Youth Mental Health: The U.S. Surgeon General's Advisory. Office of the U.S. Surgeon General. Retrieved from: https://www.hhs.gov/sites/default/files/sg-youth-mental-health-social-media-advisory.pdf

63. O'Donnell, B. (2021). "Rise in online enticement and other trends: NCMEC releases 2020 exploitation stats." Retrieved from: https://www.missingkids.org/blog/2021/rise-in-online-enticement-and-other-trends--ncmec-releases-2020-.

64. Pew Research Center (2020). "The Virtues and Downsides of Online Dating." Retrieved from: https://www.pewresearch.org/fact-tank/2020/02/06/10-facts-about-americans-and-online-dating/.

65. National Intimate Partner and Sexual Violence Survey (2021). Centers for Disease Control and Prevention. Retrieved from: https://www.cdc.gov/injury/features/prevent-stalking/index.html.

66. Pew Research Center. "The Virtues and Downsides of Online Dating."

67. Fritz, N., Malic, V., Paul, B., and Zhou, Y. (2021). "Worse than objects: The depiction of black women and men and their sexual relationship in pornography." *Gender Issues* 38(1): 100–120.

68. Zhou, Y., and Paul, B. (2016). "Lotus blossom or dragon lady: A content analysis of 'Asian women' online pornography." *Sexuality & Culture* 20(4): 1083–1100; Fritz, N., et al. "Worse than objects."

69. Pornhub Tech Review (2021). Retrieved from: https://www.pornhub.com/insights/tech-review.

70. These questions have been adapted from NAMLE's "Key Questions to Ask When Analyzing Media Messages." Retrieved on June 12, 2022 from: https://namle.net/wp-content/uploads/2021/06/Key-Questions.pdf.

71. Cho, C. H., and Cheon, H. J. (2005). "Children's exposure to negative Internet content: Effects of family context." *Journal of Broadcasting & Electronic Media* 49(4): 488–509; Byrne, S., Katz, S. J., Lee, T., Linz, D., and McIlrath, M. (2014). "Peers, predators, and porn: Predicting

parental underestimation of children's risky online experiences." *Journal of Computer-Mediated Communication* 19(2): 215–231; Wisniewski, P., Xu, H., Rosson, M. B., and Carroll, J. M. (February 2017). "Parents just don't understand: Why teens don't talk to parents about their online risk experiences." In *Proceedings of the 2017 ACM conference on computer supported cooperative work and social computing*: 523–540.

72. Fritz, N., Paul, B., Dodge, B., Fortenberry, J. D., and Herbenick, D. (2022). "Porn sex versus real sex: Sexual behaviors reported by a U.S. probability survey compared to depictions of sex in mainstream Internet-based pornography." *Archives of Sexual Behavior* 51(2): 1187–1200.

73. Bridges, A. J., Wosnitzer, R., Scharrer, E., Sun, C., and Liberman, R. (2010). "Aggression and sexual behavior in best-selling pornography videos: A content analysis update." *Violence against women* 16(10): 1065–1085; Fritz, N., Malic, V., Paul, B., and Zhou, Y. (2020). "A descriptive analysis of the types, targets, and relative frequency of aggression in mainstream pornography." *Archives of Sexual Behavior* 49(8): 3041–3053; Willis, M., Canan, S. N., Jozkowski, K. N., and Bridges, A. J. (2020). "Sexual consent communication in best-selling pornography films: A content analysis." *Journal of Sex Research* 57(1): 52–63.

74. Tholander, M., Johansson, S., Thunell, K., and Dahlström, Ö. (2022). "Traces of pornography: Shame, scripted action, and agency in narratives of young Swedish women." *Sexuality & Culture* 26: 1–21.

75. Armstrong, E. A., England, P., and Fogarty, A. C. K. (2012). "Accounting for women's orgasm and sexual enjoyment in college hookups and relationships." *American Sociological Review* 77(3): 435–462.

76. Underwood, J. M., Brener, N., Thornton, J., et al. (2020). "Youth Risk Behavior Surveillance System—United States," 2019. *MMWR Suppl 2020* 69(1): 1–83.

77. Lindberg, L. D., Scott, R. H., Desai, S., and Pleasure, Z. H. (2021). "Comparability of estimates and trends in adolescent sexual and contraceptive behaviors from two national surveys: National Survey of Family Growth and the Youth Risk Behavior Survey." *PLOS One* 16(7): e0253262; Herbenick, D., Reece, M., Sanders, S. A., Schick, V., Dodge, B., and Fortenberry, J. D. (2010). "Sexual behavior in the United States:

Results from a national probability sample of males and females ages 14 to 94." *Journal of Sexual Medicine 7* (suppl 5): 255–265.

78. Tholander, M., Johansson, S., Thunell, K., and Dahlström, Ö. (2022). "Traces of pornography: Shame, scripted action, and agency in narratives of young Swedish women." *Sexuality & Culture 26*: 1–21.

79. Keene, S. (2021). "Just fantasy? Online pornography's contribution to experiences of harm." In *The Emerald International Handbook of Technology-Facilitated Violence and Abuse* (pp. 289–308). Emerald Publishing Limited; Rothman, E. F., Kaczmarsky, C., Burke, N., Jansen, E., and Baughman, A. (2015). "'Without porn . . . I wouldn't know half the things I know now': A qualitative study of pornography use among a sample of urban, low-income, Black and Hispanic youth." *Journal of Sex Research 52*(7): 736–746; Vera Cruz, G., and Sheridan, T. (2022). "The normalization of violence during sex among young Mozambicans reportedly under the influence of pornography." *Sexuality & Culture 26*(1): 397–417; Tholander, M., et al. "Traces of Pornography."

80. Herbenick, D., Reece, M., Sanders, S. A., Schick, V., Dodge, B., and Fortenberry, J. D. (2010). "Sexual behavior in the United States: Results from a national probability sample of males and females ages 14 to 94." *Journal of Sexual Medicine 7* (suppl 5): 255–265.

81. Herbenick, D., et al., "Sexual diversity in the United States."

82. Fahs, B., and Gonzalez, J. (2014). "The front lines of the 'back door': Navigating (dis) engagement, coercion, and pleasure in women's anal sex experiences." *Feminism & Psychology 24*(4): 500–520; Faustino, M. J., and Gavey, N. (2021). "'You feel like normal sex is not enough anymore': Women's experiences of coercive and unwanted anal sex with men." *Violence Against Women 28*(11): 2624–2648.

83. Herbenick, D., Schick, V., Sanders, S. A., Reece, M., and Fortenberry, J. D. (2015). "Pain experienced during vaginal and anal intercourse with other-sex partners: Findings from a nationally representative probability study in the United States." *Journal of Sexual Medicine 12*(4): 1040–1051.

84. Jozkowski, K. N., and Peterson, Z. D. (2013). "College students and sexual consent: Unique insights." *Journal of Sex Research 50*(6): 517–523.

85. Herbenick, D., Fu, T. C., Wright, P., Paul, B., Gradus, R., Bauer, J., and Jones, R. (2020). "Diverse sexual behaviors and pornography use: Findings from a nationally representative probability survey of Americans aged 18 to 60 years." *Journal of Sexual Medicine 17*(4): 623–633.

86. Kort, J. (February 2016). "Guys on the side: Looking beyond gay tops and bottoms." Huffington Post. Retrieved from: https://www.huffpost .com/entry/guys-on-the-side-looking-beyond-gay-tops-and-bottoms _b_3082484.

87. Magnusson, L. (2020). "Unga har inte fått lära sig det viktigaste med sex." *Dagens Nyheter*. Retrieved from: https://www.dn.se/ledare/lisa -magnusson-unga-har-inte-fatt-lara-sig-det-viktigaste-med-sex/.

88. Fulbright, Y. K. (2022). "Should sex educators talk about choking during sex?" *Psychology Today*. Retrieved from: https://www.psychologytoday .com/ie/blog/mate-relate-and-communicate/202201/should-sex -educators-talk-about-choking-during-sex.

89. Vera Cruz, G., and Sheridan, T. (2022). "The normalization of violence during sex among young Mozambicans reportedly under the influence of pornography." *Sexuality & Culture 26*(1): 397–417; Rothman, E. F., et al. "'Without porn . . . I wouldn't know half the things I know now.'"

90. Sprott, R. A., and Benoit Hadcock, B. (2018). "Bisexuality, pansexuality, queer identity, and kink identity." *Sexual and Relationship Therapy 33*(1–2): 214–232.

91. Burch, R. L., and Salmon, C. (2019). "The rough stuff: Understanding aggressive consensual sex." *Evolutionary Psychological Science 5*(4): 383–393. Herbenick, D., Fu, T. C., Valdivia, D. S., Patterson, C., Gonzalez, Y. R., Guerra-Reyes, L., Eastman-Mueller, H., Beckmeyer, J., and Rosenberg, M. (2021). "What is rough sex, who does it, and who likes it? Findings from a probability sample of US undergraduate students." *Archives of Sexual Behavior 50*: 1183–1195.

92. Herbenick, D., Patterson, C., Beckmeyer, J., Rosenstock Gonzalez, Y.R., Luetke, M., Guerra-Reyes, L., Eastman-Mueller, H., Svetina Valdivia, D., and Rosenberg, M. (2021). "Diverse sexual behaviors in undergraduate students: Findings from a campus probability survey." *Journal of Sexual Medicine 18*(6): 1024–1041.

93. Surnow, R. & Hsieh, C. (2020). Face-sitting. *Cosmopolitan*. Published on December 22, 2020. Retrieved on June 7, 2023 from: https://www.cosmopolitan.com/sexopedia/a8271867/facesitting-definition/.

94. Burch, R. L., and Salmon, C. (2022). "Rough sex and pornography preferences: Novelty seeking, not aggression." *Journal of the Evolutionary Studies Consortium*. Retrieved from: http://evostudies.org/evos-journal/about-the-journal/; Beres, M. A., Pearman-Beres, L. J., and Johns, P. (2020). "Youth healthy and safe relationships: A literature review." University of Otago: New Zealand.

95. Lee, E. M., Klement, K. R., and Sagarin, B. J. (2015). "Double hanging during consensual sexual asphyxia: a response to Roma, Pazzelli, Pompili, Girardi, and Ferracuti (2013)." *Archives of Sexual Behavior 44*: 1751–1753.

96. De Boos, J. (2019). "Non-fatal strangulation: Hidden injuries, hidden risks." *Emergency Medicine Australasia 31*(3): 302–308; Lee, Klement, and Sagarin. "Double hanging during consensual sexual asphyxia."

97. Valera, E. M., Colantonio, A., Daugherty, J. C., Scott, O. C., and Berenbaum, H. (2022). "Strangulation as an acquired brain injury in intimate-partner violence and its relationship to cognitive and psychological functioning: A preliminary study." *Journal of Head Trauma Rehabilitation 37*(1): 15–23.

98. Hou, J., Huibregtse, M., Alexander, I. L., Klemsz, L. M., Fu, T. C., Fortenberry, J. D., Herbenick, D., and Kawata, K. (In press). "Association of frequent sexual choking/strangulation with neurophysiological responses: A pilot resting-state fMRI study." *Journal of Neurotrauma*; Huibregtse, M. E., Alexander, I. L., Klemsz, L. M., Fu, T. C., Fortenberry, J. D., Herbenick, D., and Kawata, K. (2022). "Frequent and recent non-fatal strangulation/choking during sex and its association with fMRI activation during working memory tasks." *Frontiers in Behavioral Neuroscience 16*: 881678.

99. Brennan, D. (2021). "What is sexual asphyxiation?" WebMD. Retrieved from: https://www.webmd.com/sex/what-is-sexual-asphyxiation.

100. "Want to know more about rough sex and choking?" The Light Project. Retrieved on February 20, 2023 from: https://www.intheknow.co.nz/rough-sex-and-choking.

101. Newmahr, S. (2010). "Rethinking kink: Sadomasochism as serious leisure." *Qualitative Sociology 33*: 313–331; Brennan, "What is sexual asphyxiation?"

102. Lewis, L. F., Ward, C., Jarvis, N., and Cawley, E. (2021). "'Straight sex is complicated enough!': The lived experiences of autistics who are gay, lesbian, bisexual, asexual, or other sexual orientations." *Journal of Autism and Developmental Disorders 51*(7): 2324–2337; Bush, H. H., Williams, L. W., and Mendes, E. (2021). "Brief report: Asexuality and young women on the autism spectrum." *Journal of Autism and Developmental Disorders 51*(2): 725–733.

103. Brown-Lavoie, S. M., Viecili, M. A., and Weiss, J. (2014). "Sexual knowledge and victimization in adults with autism spectrum disorders." *Journal of Autism and Developmental Disorders 44*(9): 2185–2196.

104. Ballan, M. S. (2012). "Parental perspectives of communication about sexuality in families of children with autism spectrum disorders." *Journal of Autism and Developmental Disorders 42*(5): 676–684.

105. Mintah, K., and Parlow, S. E. (2018). "Are you flirting with me? Autistic traits, theory of mind, and inappropriate courtship." *Personality and Individual Differences 128*: 100–106.

106. Mogavero, M. C., and Hsu, K. H. (2020). "Dating and courtship behaviors among those with autism spectrum disorder." *Sexuality and Disability 38*(2): 355–364.

107. Bertilsdotter Rosqvist, H., and Jackson-Perry, D. (2021). "Not doing it properly? (Re) producing and resisting knowledge through narratives of autistic sexualities." *Sexuality and Disability 39*(2): 327–344; Gray, S., Kirby, A. V., and Graham Holmes, L. (2021). "Autistic Narratives of Sensory Features, Sexuality, and Relationships." *Autism in Adulthood 3*(3): 238–246; Bauer, R. (2008). "Transgressive and transformative gendered sexual practices and white privileges: The case of the dyke/trans BDSM communities." *Women's Studies Quarterly 36*(3/4): 233–253.

INDEX

ABOUT THE AUTHOR

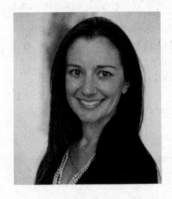

Debby Herbenick, PhD, is an award-winning, internationally recognized sexuality researcher and an AASECT-certified sexuality educator. She is a Provost Professor at the Indiana University School of Public Health and the author of five bestselling books about human sexuality. Dr. Herbenick is the lead investigator of the National Survey of Sexual Health and Behavior, which has tracked sexual trends in the United States since 2009. Dr. Herbenick has been published in the *Washington Post*, *New York Times*, *Men's Health* magazine, and *Glamour*, among others, and she has provided expert opinions about sex on television shows such as *Tyra*, *Katie*, *The Doctors*, and *The Tamron Hall Show*. She was born and raised in Miami, Florida, and now lives in Bloomington, Indiana.

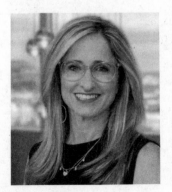

Susan Stone, Esq., has dedicated her life to helping students in crisis and meeting their legal needs. As cochair of the Student & Athlete Defense group at KJK law firm in Cleveland, Ohio, Susan handles matters ranging from special education issues to student disciplinary matters and Title IX investigations, and has gained a national reputation for representing students and professors in Title IX cases. Susan is certified in restorative justice, and has also guided students through informal resolution, including mediation and restorative justice. In addition, Susan proudly cohosts the podcast *Real Talk with Susan and Kristina* to discuss with outside guests cutting-edge issues affecting students.

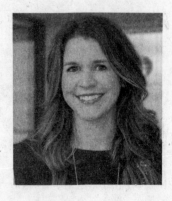

Kristina Supler advocates for students of all ages during the most difficult periods in their lives. Her experience is regularly enlisted for cases involving reports of sexual assault, and her services are particularly sought after to navigate complex Title IX cases with a parallel criminal investigation. Kristina also helps students facing academic integrity violations and other types of student discipline. She recognizes the emotional toll that cases take on families, and she brings empathy to her work. Kristina understands the importance of alternative forms of dispute resolution in a variety of contexts. Given the breadth of her legal experience, Kristina regularly writes and speaks on issues involving students and education.